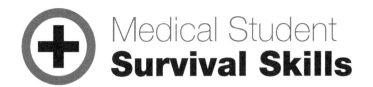

Medical Student
Survival Skills

History Taking and Communication Skills

T0261903

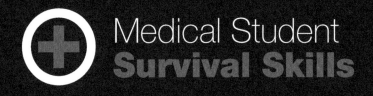

Medical Student
Survival Skills

History Taking and Communication Skills

Philip Jevon RN BSc(Hons) PGCE
Academy Manager/Tutor
Walsall Teaching Academy, Manor Hospital, Walsall, UK

Steve Odogwu FRCS
Consultant, General Surgery, Senior Academy Tutor
Walsall Teaching Academy, Manor Hospital, Walsall, UK

Consulting Editors

Jonathan Pepper BMedSci BM BS FRCOG
MD FAcadMEd
Consultant Obstetrics and Gynaecology, Head of Academy
Walsall Healthcare NHS Trust, Manor Hospital, Walsall, UK

Jamie Coleman MBChB MD MA(Med Ed) FRCP FBPhS
Professor in Clinical Pharmacology and Medical Education / MBChB Deputy
   Programme Director
School of Medicine, University of Birmingham, Birmingham, UK

WILEY Blackwell

This edition first published 2020
© 2020 by John Wiley & Sons Ltd

The right of Philip Jevon and Steve Odogwu to be identified as the authors in this work has been asserted in accordance with law.

Registered Office(s)
John Wiley & Sons, Inc., 111 River Street, Hoboken, NJ 07030, USA
John Wiley & Sons Ltd, The Atrium, Southern Gate, Chichester, West Sussex, PO19 8SQ, UK

Editorial Office
9600 Garsington Road, Oxford, OX4 2DQ, UK

For details of our global editorial offices, customer services, and more information about Wiley products visit us at www.wiley.com.

Wiley also publishes its books in a variety of electronic formats and by print-on-demand. Some content that appears in standard print versions of this book may not be available in other formats.

Library of Congress Cataloging-in-Publication Data
Names: Jevon, Philip, author. | Odogwu, Steve, author.
Title: Medical student survival skills. History taking and communication skills / Philip Jevon, Steve Odogwu.
Other titles: History taking and communication skills
Description: Hoboken, NJ : Wiley-Blackwell, 2020. | Includes index. |
Identifiers: LCCN 2018060341 (print) | LCCN 2018060741 (ebook) | ISBN 9781118862704
  (Adobe PDF) | ISBN 9781118862698 (ePub) | ISBN 9781118862681 (pbk.)
Subjects: | MESH: Medical History Taking–methods | Professional-Patient Relations | Handbook
Classification: LCC R118 (ebook) | LCC R118 (print) | NLM WB 39 | DDC 610.1/4–dc23
LC record available at https://lccn.loc.gov/2018060341

Cover Design: Wiley
Cover Image: © WonderfulPixel/Shutterstock

Set in 9.25/12.5pt Helvetica Neue by SPi Global, Pondicherry, India

Printed in Great Britain by TJ International Ltd, Padstow, Cornwall

10 9 8 7 6 5 4 3 2 1

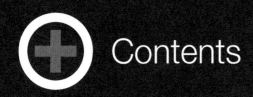 Contents

Acknowledgements

We are very grateful for the following doctors, most of who were based at the Manor Hospital in Walsall, for their help with the manuscript.

Part 1: History Taking

Abdominal distention	Dr. Prashant Patel
Abdominal pain in pregnancy	Dr. Chloe Ross
Abdominal pain	Dr. Michael ding
Alcohol intake	Dr. Manisha Choudhary
Amenorrhoea	Dr. Beth-Anne Garman
Anxiety	Dr. Tracy Hancox
Ataxia	Dr. Nevan Meghani
Back pain	Dr. Salina Ali
Chest pain	Dr. Sanam Anwari
Collapse and loss of conciousness	Dr. Amar Lally
Confusion	Dr. Nicola Lowe
Constipation	Dr. Jess Chang
Cough	Dr. Knapp Claire
Deliberate self-harm	Dr. Nicola Lowe
Diarrhoea	Dr. S Mensforth & C McMahon
Dizziness and vertigo	Dr. Halimah Alazzani
Dyspepsia	Dr. Halimah Alazzani
Dysphagia	Dr. Imad Adwan
Dysphasia	Dr. Halimah Alazzani
Dysuria	Dr. Manisha Choudhary
Otalgia – ear ache	Dr. Karan Jolly
Falls	Dr. Sarah Mensforth
Fever	Dr. Beth-Anne Garman
Haematemesis	Dr. Imad Adwan
Haematuria	Dr. Dominic Williams & Dr. Seshagiri Thirukkatigavoor

Haemoptysis	Dr. Sanam Anwari
Headache	Dr. Amar Lally
Hoarseness	Dr. Karan Jolly
Jaundice	Dr. Jennifer Hardy
Joint pain	Dr. Jon Catley
Acute leg pain (ischaemic leg)	Dr. Ayaz Vanta
Leg ulcer	Dr. Oliver Oxenham
Loin pain	Dr. Mohammed Jamil Aslam
Loss of memory	Dr. Amy Burlingham
Low mood	Dr. Tracy Hancox
Lumps and bumps	Dr. Salman Waqar
Melaena	Dr. Jess Chang
Menorrhagia	Dr. Tracy Hancox
Nausea	Dr. Sameer Patel
Numbness and weakness	Dr. Halimah Alazzani
Paediatrics: Diarrhoea	Dr. Chloe Ross
Paediatrics: Convulsions/seizures	Dr. Chloe Ross
Paediatrics: Difficulty in breathing	Dr. Chloe Ross
Paediatrics: Non-specific unwell neonate	Dr. Chloe Ross
Paediatrics: Vomiting	Dr. Chloe Ross
Paediatrics: Wheeze	Dr. Chloe Ross
Pain	Dr. Jennifer Hardy & Dr. Katie Ramm
Palpitations	Dr. Sameer Patel
Paresthesia	Dr. Nevan Meghani
Per rectum bleeding	Dr. Jess Chang
Preoperative assessment	Dr. Gagandeep Panesar
Per vaginum bleeding in pregnancy	Dr. Tracy Hancox
Pruritus	Dr. Seow Li-Fay
Pervaginal bleed	Dr. Emily Tabb
Pervaginal discharge	Dr. Chloe Ross
Rash	Dr. Seow Li-Fay
Red eye – Painless	Dr. Rohit Jolly
Red eye – Painful	Dr. Rohit Jolly
Seizure	Dr. Amit Rajput

About the companion website

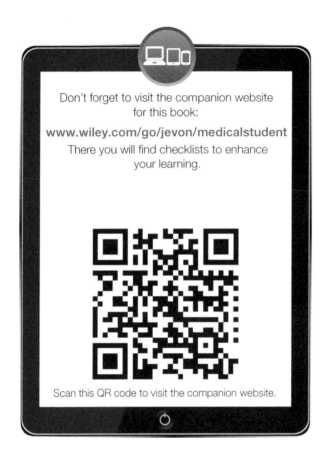

Don't forget to visit the companion website for this book:

www.wiley.com/go/jevon/medicalstudent

There you will find checklists to enhance your learning.

Scan this QR code to visit the companion website.

Part 1

History Taking

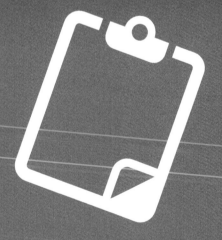

① Abdominal distention

Definition: Abdominal distension is a sense of increased abdominal pressure that involves an actual measurable change in the circumference of a person's abdomen.

Differentials

- *Common* (important causes): ascites, bowel obstruction (from cancer, adhesions, sigmoid volvulus, hernia, etc.), diverticulitis, coeliac disease, inflammatory bowel disease (IBD), constipation, medications

History

 NB Infection control measures.

History of presenting complaint
- Open question assessing duration of abdominal distention
- Onset, triggers, how long for
- When was the last time they opened their bowels/passed wind. If they can open their bowels, does this relieve the distention?
- Any per rectum (PR) bleeding
- Any vomiting/nausea
- Abdominal pain: use SOCRATES template (see Chapter 8)
- Any weight loss
- Any change in appetite
- Any shortness of breath
- Previous abdominal distention

Medical Student Survival Skills: History Taking and Communication Skills, First Edition.
Philip Jevon and Steve Odogwu.
© 2020 John Wiley & Sons Ltd. Published 2020 by John Wiley & Sons Ltd.
Companion website: www.wiley.com/go/jevon/medicalstudent

3

- Any signs of jaundice – pale stools, dark urine, itching
- Urine symptoms: dysuria/frequency/dribbling/hesitation, etc.

Past medical and surgical history
- Constipation, diarrhoea, change in bowel habit. Any IBD?
- Any previous surgery, especially gynaecological/abdominal
- Any previous medical history
- Use MJ THREADS (Box 1.1)

Box 1.1 MJ THREADS	
M	Myocardial infarction
J	Jaundice
T	Tuberculosis
H	Hypertension ('Has anyone told you, you have high blood pressure?')
R	Rheumatic fever
E	Epilepsy
A	Asthma
D	Diabetes
S	Stroke

Medications and allergies
- Current medications
- Allergies

Family history
- Any family members with similar symptoms
- Any family history of malignancy
- Any illnesses that run in the family

Social history
- Who patient lives with
- Occupation (e.g. healthcare setting)
- Smoking and alcohol
- Recent foreign travel

OSCE Key Learning Points

✔ In particular, be aware of bowel obstruction and ascites. Do not forget vomiting, last open bowels, and weight loss

Investigations

- *Bloods*: full blood count (FBC), urea and electrolytes (U&Es), C-reactive protein (CRP), amylase, clotting, albumin, international normalised ratio (INR)
- *Imaging*:
  - *Erect chest X-ray – perforation/pleural effusion*
  - *Abdominal X-ray – bowel obstruction/toxic megacolon (for ulcerative colitis)*
  - *Computed tomograpy (CT) of the abdomen – to further investigate the cause of, for* example, bowel obstruction/ascites
- *Diagnostic/therapeutic*: ascitic tap if presence of ascites – transudate or exudate

2 Abdominal pain in pregnancy

> **Definition:** Pain in the abdominal area whilst pregnant (this chapter is aimed at later pregnancy of ≥ 20 weeks and does not involve early pregnancy causes such as miscarriage and ectopic pregnancy).

Differentials

- *Common*: urinary tract infection (UTI), constipation, symphysis pubis dysfunction, ligament stretching, labour, placental abruption, pre-eclampsia, surgical causes (including appendicitis and cholecystitis), pyelonephritis, ovarian cyst torsion/rupture, uterine fibroid torsion or red degeneration
- *Rare*: uterine rupture, uterine torsion, rectus sheath haematoma, acute fatty liver of pregnancy

History

 NB Pregnant women are still prone to conditions that cause abdominal pain in non-pregnant women, read in conjunction with Chapter 3.

History of presenting complaint
- What is the abdominal pain like – use the SOCRATES approach (see Chapter 8)
- Any per vaginum (PV) bleeding? If so quantify amount, number of episodes and type of blood
- Are they feeling the baby move ok?
- Any change in discharge or episode of watery discharge
- Any nausea or vomiting

Medical Student Survival Skills: History Taking and Communication Skills, First Edition.
Philip Jevon and Steve Odogwu.
© 2020 John Wiley & Sons Ltd. Published 2020 by John Wiley & Sons Ltd.
Companion website: www.wiley.com/go/jevon/medicalstudent

- Any dysuria or frequency or retention
- Are the bowels open normally; any constipation or diarrhoea
- Any headache or blurred vision
- Any swelling
- Any fevers
- Any jaundice
- When was the last time they had fluid and/or food (in case they need to go to theatre)?

Past medical and surgical history
- Obstetric history
  - Current gestation
  - Number of previous pregnancies including miscarriages, terminations, and still births and gestations and types of these (e.g. medical or surgical termination, was it a missed miscarriage and required medical or surgical treatment?)
  - Number of live births – gestation, mode of delivery, any problems during pregnancy, with the labour or with the child
  - For this pregnancy – any problems so far, any problems on scans, any hospital admissions
- Any medical conditions – any known fibroids, ovarian cysts, congenital uterine abnormalities
- Any operations – particularly gynaecological or abdominal

Medications and allergies
- Any regular medications, any recent medications
- Any allergies

Family history
- Any family history of pre-eclampsia

Social history
- Who lives at home
- Occupation
- Smoking – number per day and for how many years
- Alcohol – number of units per week

OSCE Key Learning Points

✔ Appendicitis in pregnancy can present with more generalised abdominal pain or at times right upper quadrant (RUQ) pain, and guarding and rebound tenderness are less pronounced

✔ Degree of abdominal pain and bleeding is not related to degree of placental abruption

 Common misinterpretations and pitfalls

Remember to consider non-obstetric causes of abdominal pain. Always check well-being of the mother and baby (ask about foetal movements).

3 Abdominal pain

Definition: Pain felt in the abdomen.

Differentials

- *Common*: urinary tract infections (UTIs), appendicitis, gastroenteritis (viral, bacterial, and parasitic), ulcers, inflammatory bowel disease (IBD), constipation, gallstones, cholecystitis, pancreatitis, pelvic inflammatory disease, kidney stones, bowel cancer, irritable bowel syndrome (IBS), mesenteric adenitis, diverticulitis
- *Rare*: coeliac disease, lymphoma, abdominal aortic aneurysm (important not to miss), ectopic pregnancy, Henoch–Schonlein purpura, intussusception

History

History of presenting complaint
- Site
- Onset
- Character
- Radiation
- Associations – with food (biliary colic)
- Time course
- Exacerbating/relieving factors
- Severity
- Nausea/vomiting
- Dysphagia
- Bowels – regular, diarrhoea, constipation, bloatedness, altered bowel habit, hard to flush, tenesmus

Medical Student Survival Skills: History Taking and Communication Skills, First Edition.
Philip Jevon and Steve Odogwu.
© 2020 John Wiley & Sons Ltd. Published 2020 by John Wiley & Sons Ltd.
Companion website: www.wiley.com/go/jevon/medicalstudent

- Malaena/rectal bleeding
- Any weight loss, fever, anorexia, lethargy, or early satiety
- Jaundice
- Menstrual history – last menstrual period, regularity, contraception, pregnancy, amenorrhoea, dyspareunia, post-coital bleeding or PV bleeding/discharge
- Urinary-dysuria, frequency, hesitancy, post-micturition dribbling, haematuria, history of recurrent UTIs,

Past medical and surgical history
- Previous abdominal pains
- Constipation, diarrhoea, IBS, IBD
- Any other illnesses
- Any previous surgery – especially gynaecological or abdominal

Medications and allergies
- Current medications, laxative use, recent antibiotics
- Allergies

Family history
- Any family members with similar symptoms
- Any illnesses which run in the family, coeliac disease, IBS, IBD, malignancies

Social history
- Who patient lives with
- Occupation (e.g. healthcare setting)
- Smoking and alcohol
- Recent foreign travel

OSCE Key Learning Points

✔ In particular, remember to ask about weight loss, altered bowel habits, and bleeding

NB Any change in bowel habit, especially in the elderly, should be fully investigated.

4 Alcohol intake

History

History of presenting complaint
- Alcohol intake
- Frequency of consumption
- Units consumed per day/per week/per session (if binging)
- Adequate dietary intake
- CAGE (screening method):
  - **C**ut down on drinking
  - **A**nnoyed by criticism of drinking
  - **G**uilty about drinking
  - **E**ye opener
- Evidence of withdrawal:
  - Tremor, confusion
  - Seizures, hallucinations (delirium tremens)
- Previous rehabilitation or alcohol cessation

Past medical history
- Mental health disorders
- Liver cirrhosis, hypertension, cardiac arrhythmias
- Gastric/peptic ulcers, varices, pancreatitis

Medications and allergies
- Current medications
- Allergies

Social history
- Who patient lives with, housing
- Smoking, illicit drug use

Medical Student Survival Skills: History Taking and Communication Skills, First Edition.
Philip Jevon and Steve Odogwu.
© 2020 John Wiley & Sons Ltd. Published 2020 by John Wiley & Sons Ltd.
Companion website: www.wiley.com/go/jevon/medicalstudent

- Support network
- Social services involvement

OSCE Key Learning Points

✔ The social history is of particular importance

OSCES Key Learning Points

Units of alcohol

✔ Men should not regularly drink $>3–4$ units of alcohol per day

✔ Women should not regularly drink $>2–3$ units of alcohol per day

✔ 1 unit of alcohol: e.g. small shot of spirit

✔ 2 units of alcohol: pint of beer, can of lager, or standard glass of wine

✔ 3 units of alcohol: large glass of wine or pint of strong lager

(Source: www.nhs.uk)

5 Amenorrhoea

Definition: Amenorrhoea is the absence of menstruation. There are two classifications:
- *Primary* if menstruation not started by age 16 years
- *Secondary* if previously normal menstruation has stopped for more than 6 months

NB Oligomenorrhoea is when menstruation occurs every 35 days to 6 months.

Differentials

- *Common*:
  - Physiological – pregnancy, lactation, post-menopausal, constitutional delay
  - Pathological – premature menopause (<40 years), polycystic ovarian syndrome, hyperprolactinaemia, stress
- *Rare*: Turner's syndrome, virilising tumours, anatomical (e.g. cervical stenosis)

NB Consider causes in the hypothalamus, pituitary, thyroid, adrenals, ovaries, uterus, or vagina.

Medical Student Survival Skills: History Taking and Communication Skills, First Edition.
Philip Jevon and Steve Odogwu.
© 2020 John Wiley & Sons Ltd. Published 2020 by John Wiley & Sons Ltd.
Companion website: www.wiley.com/go/jevon/medicalstudent

History

 Common misinterpretations and pitfalls

Remember to check if the patient could be pregnant or menopausal – amenorrhoea can be physiological.

History of presenting complaint
- Age
- Previous menstruation
- Time since last period (if relevant)
- Normal menstrual cycle – regularity, duration, frequency (if relevant)
- Presence of secondary sexual characteristics (if primary)
- Sexual activity
- Pelvic pain
- Hirsutism, acne
- Weight/body mass index (BMI) and weight loss or gain
- Exercise and eating habits
- Stressful events
- Menopausal symptoms (hot flushes, night sweats, loss of libido)
- Symptoms of thyroid disease

 NB Low BMI or excessive exercise can cause hypothalamic hypogonadism.

Past medical history
- Obstetric history
- Post-partum haemorrhage (Sheehan's syndrome)
- Hyper- or hypothyroidism
- Diabetes or insulin resistance

Past surgical history
- Any gynaecological procedure (oophorectomy, endometrial resection, ablation)
- Evacuation of retained products of conception (Asherman's syndrome)
- Thyroidectomy

Medications and allergies
- Current medications
- Contraceptives
- Antipsychotics
- Previous cytotoxics
- Allergies

 NB Antipsychotics and hypothyroidism can cause hyperprolactinaemia.

Family history
- Constitutional delay

Social history
- Smoking and alcohol

OSCE Key Learning Points

✔ Investigations include pregnancy test, thyroid function tests, hormone levels (luteinising hormone (LH), follicle stimulating hormone (FSH), gonadotrophin releasing hormone (GnRH), oestradiol, prolactin, testosterone, sex hormone binding globulin (SHBG), glucose tolerance test, lipid profile, transvaginal ultrasound (polycystic ovary syndrome), and magnetic resonance imaging (MRI) of the brain (hypothalamus/pituitary tumours)

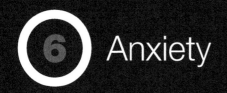

6 Anxiety

Definition: A feeling of unease or fear that is out of proportion to what would be expected.

Differentials

- *Common*: anxiety/phobic disorders, depression, secondary to physical illness
- *Rare*: medication or illicit substance side effects, other psychiatric illness (obsessive–compulsive disorder, post-traumatic stress disorder, eating disorder), endocrine (e.g. hyperthyroidism)

History

 NB Ensure your personal safety (i.e. sit nearer the door).

History of presenting complaint
- Explore anxiety: generalised anxiety, panic attacks, course of anxiety
- Any precipitating factor (e.g. military)
- Panic attacks: triggers/spontaneous, onset, physical symptoms, duration, calming strategies
- Biological symptoms: sleep, appetite, weight loss, fatigue, poor concentration, poor libido, sweating, palpitations, breathlessness, tight chest, dizziness
- Effect on their life and social functioning (e.g. due to avoidance of triggers)
- Explore for mood changes, delusions (paranoia, poverty, grandiose), hallucinations (auditory, olfactory, visual), thought disorder (insertion/withdrawal)

Medical Student Survival Skills: History Taking and Communication Skills, First Edition.
Philip Jevon and Steve Odogwu.
© 2020 John Wiley & Sons Ltd. Published 2020 by John Wiley & Sons Ltd.
Companion website: www.wiley.com/go/jevon/medicalstudent

- Pre-morbid personality (anxious personality)
- Enquire about other physical symptoms (of endocrine disease, unexplained symptoms)
- Ask about current thoughts or plans of self-harm/suicide
- Ask about thought or plans to harm others and any relevant forensic history

Past medical and surgical history
- Any concurrent illnesses (acute or chronic)
- Past psychiatric history (secondary psychiatric input, psychological therapies)
- Previous self-harm/suicide attempts
- If time; could explore personal history and childhood

Medications and allergies
- Current medications, anxiolytics
- Allergies

Family history
- Any family members with similar symptoms
- Any psychiatric illnesses in relatives

Social history
- Who patient lives with (supportive partner/domestic abuse/are they a carer?)
- Smoking, alcohol and drug misuse
- Social coping strategies
- Children (safeguarding)
- Occupation (stress/sick leave), hobbies, other responsibilities

OSCE Key Learning Points

✔ In particular, do not forget to ask about thoughts and history of self-harm, suicide, and harm to others

 NB Anxiety often presents concomitantly with other psychiatric illness, depression, other neuroses, substance misuse, or personality disorder.

Uncommon presentations

Anxiety can present in many forms. Be mindful of anxiety and stress in a patient who presents frequently with seemingly trivial medical complaints, or often misses appointments.

 Common misinterpretations and pitfalls

Anxiety is common, a feeling that everyone has from time to time. To be clinically important it should affect the patient's life and well-being.

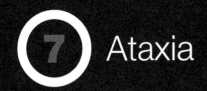 Ataxia

Definition: Ataxia is a neurological sign consisting of uncoordinated or clumsy muscle movements that is not the result of muscle weakness. The term is often used to describe a person's gait. It can be caused by cerebellar, vestibular, or proprioceptive (sensory) dysfunction.

Differentials

- *Cerebellar and vestibular*: e.g. focal lesions such as stroke and brain tumour
- *Sensory*: e.g. peripheral neuropathy

History

History of presenting complaint
- Onset of symptoms
- Duration of symptoms
- When the symptoms occur
- Pain – difficulty walking may be due to pain or compensation for weakness of a single muscle group
- Associated symptoms – will give clues to the cause of ataxia
  - Cerebellar – risk factors and positive findings on cerebellar examination will guide diagnosis
  - Sensory – risk factors, characteristic 'stomping' gait, and Romberg's test will guide diagnosis
  - Vestibular – coexisting vertigo, nausea, and vomiting suggest vestibular causes

Past medical and surgical history
- Previous cancer?
- Previous head trauma?

Medical Student Survival Skills: History Taking and Communication Skills, First Edition.
Philip Jevon and Steve Odogwu.
© 2020 John Wiley & Sons Ltd. Published 2020 by John Wiley & Sons Ltd.
Companion website: www.wiley.com/go/jevon/medicalstudent

- Cardiovascular risk factors – hypertension, hypercholesterolaemia, smoking, diabetes
- Diabetes control
- Any other illnesses
- Previous brain or spinal surgery

Medications and allergies
- Current and previous medications
- Allergies

Social history
- Alcohol – important to look for current or previous alcohol excess
- Diet – malnutrition, vegan diet
- Drug abuse
- Occupation

Family history
- Relatives with similar symptoms – important to screen for inherited causes of ataxia

OSCE Key Learning Points

✔ Ataxia is primarily a diagnosis elicited on examination, but a thorough history will help to guide you to the correct diagnosis, by giving you the likely cause

 Common misinterpretations and pitfalls

In reality the causes of an ataxia may be multifactorial and so it is important to investigate all possible causes in order to find the correct diagnosis for these incredibly disabling symptoms. The picture may also be complicated by muscle weakness of any cause, Parkinson's disease, or frontal lobe dysfunction, which can mimic true ataxia.

8 Back pain

Differentials

- *Common*: degenerative (osteoarthritis, spondylolisthesis), trauma, wedge fractures (secondary to osteoporosis), disc prolapse, muscular, others: renal colic, endometriosis, pelvic inflammatory disease
- *Rare*: ankylosing spondylitis, abdominal aortic aneurysm, infections, e.g. tuberculosis (TB), osteomyelitis
- *Sinister*: malignancy, cord compression

 NB Always consider non-orthopaedic/rheumatological causes.

History

History of present complaint
- Pain history – use the SOCRATES approach
    - **S**ite of the pain – according to spinal anatomy (cervical, thoracic, lumbar, sacral)
    - **O**nset– acute, subacute, chronic
    - **C**haracter – sharp, dull, shooting
    - **R**adiation – to arms/legs/buttocks/neck/groin
    - **A**ssociations – numbness, paraesthesia, stiffness
    - **T**ime course – is the pain better/worse at any times of the day
    - **E**xacerbating/relieving factors – lying down, bending forwards, exercise
    - **S**everity – out of 10
- Red flag symptoms:
    - Thoracic pain
    - Night pain
    - Weight loss

Medical Student Survival Skills: History Taking and Communication Skills, First Edition.
Philip Jevon and Steve Odogwu.
© 2020 John Wiley & Sons Ltd. Published 2020 by John Wiley & Sons Ltd.
Companion website: www.wiley.com/go/jevon/medicalstudent

- Night sweats
- Numbness/weakness of limbs
- Incontinence of urine/stool
- Sacral numbness
- Recent trauma/injury
- Have they noticed an abdominal mass
- Any pain in any other joints
- Any systemic symptoms

OSCE Key Learning Points

✔ Always ask about red flags and history of malignancy

Past medical history
- Arthritis
- Any malignancies – particularly those which may cause bone metastases
- Known renal stones
- Gynaecological conditions

Family history
- Arthritis
- Malignancies

Drug history
- Long-term steroid use
- Immunosuppressants
- Is the patient on any agents for bone protection
- What analgesia do they use

Social history
- Occupation
- Social activities/hobbies
- Smoking and alcohol

 Common misinterpretations and pitfalls

Do not assume all back pain is mechanical. All other causes must be excluded.

26

9 Chest pain

Definition: Pain or discomfort that can be felt in the chest.

Differentials

- *Common*: angina/myocardial infarction, pulmonary embolism, pneumothorax, pneumonia, reflux oesophagitis
- *Rare*: aortic dissection, pericarditis

History

History of presenting complaint
- Site: retrosternal, peripheral
- Onset: sudden, gradual, triggers – on exertion, after food, on coughing, deep inspiration
- Character: constricting, sharp, central crushing pain
- Radiations: shoulder/arms, neck/jaw, epigastrium
- Associations: shortness of breath, nausea/vomiting, sweat, chest wall tenderness, palpitations, cough
- Relieving factors: rest, glyceryl trinitrate (GTN), antacids, leaning forward

Past medical and surgical history
- Previous history of chest pain
- Any other illnesses – diabetes, hypertension, hypercholesterolaemia
- Previous surgery – coronary artery bypass graft

Medications and allergies
- Current medications: non-steroidal anti-inflammatory drugs (NSAIDs), combined oral contraceptive pill (COCP), GTN, over the counter (OTC) antacids
- Allergies

Medical Student Survival Skills: History Taking and Communication Skills, First Edition.
Philip Jevon and Steve Odogwu.
© 2020 John Wiley & Sons Ltd. Published 2020 by John Wiley & Sons Ltd.
Companion website: www.wiley.com/go/jevon/medicalstudent

Family history
- Coronary artery disease, diabetes, hypertension, dyslipidaemia, congenital heart disease

Social history
- Smoking and alcohol
- Diet
- Who patient lives with
- Occupation

OSCE Key Learning Points

✔ In particular, remember to ask about the character of pain and any associations as this will often point to the cause

 NB Initial treatment of cardiac-sounding chest pain – nitrates, aspirin, clopidogrel, and enoxaparin ($1\,mg\,kg^{-1}$).

 Common misinterpretations and pitfalls

Use open-ended questions when asking about the character of pain, do not put words in the patient's mouth.

10 Collapse and loss of conciousness

Differentials

- *Common*: postural hypotension, syncope, arrhythmia, hypoglycaemia, myocardial infarction, epilepsy
- *Rare*: aortic dissection, subarachnoid haemorrhage, meningitis, pulmonary embolism

History

History of presenting complaint
- *Before the episode*
  - What were they doing at the time?
  - Warning symptoms
  - Chest pain, sweating, vomiting, palpitations
  - Abdominal pain with radiation to back/interscapular area
  - Shortness of breath, palpitations, pleuritic pain, haemoptysis
  - Neck stiffness, photophobia, headache, rash
  - Hunger, feeling faint, confusion
- *During the episode*
  - Do you remember what happened?
  - How long did it last?
  - Convulsions, tongue biting, urinary/faecal incontinence, frothing at the mouth
  - Hit their head
  - Loss of consciousness (LOC)
  - Did anybody witness the event?
- *After the episode*
  - Drowsy, confusion, amnesia, muscle aching
  - How long did it take before you felt back to normal?

Medical Student Survival Skills: History Taking and Communication Skills, First Edition.
Philip Jevon and Steve Odogwu.
© 2020 John Wiley & Sons Ltd. Published 2020 by John Wiley & Sons Ltd.
Companion website: www.wiley.com/go/jevon/medicalstudent

Past medical and surgical history
- Previous similar episodes
- Any other illnesses
- Any recent surgery

Medications and allergies
- Current medications: use of antihypertensive/diabetic medications
- Allergies

Family history
- Cardiac problems
- Any sudden deaths in the family
- Any illnesses that run in the family

Social history
- Who patient lives with
- Occupation
- Smoking and alcohol
- Driving

OSCE Key Learning Points

✔ In particular, do not forget to ask about:
✔ Collateral history
✔ If they hit their head
✔ Convulsions, tongue biting, incontinence

⑪ Confusion

The main point to clarify in the history is whether this is chronic confusion (more often a dementia) or acute confusion (more likely to have an underlying organic cause). There may also be an increase in confusion in a chronically confused patient 'acute on chronic confusion'.

Differentials

- *Common*: *chronic* – dementia; *acute* – alcohol, medications, infection, intracranial event
- *Rare*: *chronic* – endocrine and metabolic disorders, hereditary disorders; *acute* – trauma, psychosis

History

 NB Introduce yourself, try to interview in a calm environment. Gain a collaborative history.

History of presenting complaint
- Onset of symptoms – chronic or acute
- Fluctuation in symptoms
- Level of consciousness
- Assess cognitive function – Mini Mental State Examination (MMSE) or Abbreviated Mental Test (AMT)
- Hallucinations and delusions – are they reacting to stimuli which are not present or have any beliefs which are not true?
- Ask about all other physical symptoms, – i.e. 'systems review', to elicit any possible organic cause, especially dysuria, chest symptoms, and fever

Medical Student Survival Skills: History Taking and Communication Skills, First Edition.
Philip Jevon and Steve Odogwu.
© 2020 John Wiley & Sons Ltd. Published 2020 by John Wiley & Sons Ltd.
Companion website: www.wiley.com/go/jevon/medicalstudent

- Functional state – needs help with activities of daily living
- Behavioural – are there any aggressive/behavioural issues

Past medical and surgical history
- All chronic medical conditions
- Cardiovascular risk factors – can predispose to cerebral vascular accidents and vascular dementia
- Psychiatric history

Medications and allergies
- Benzodiazepines
- Anticholinergics
- Antidepressants
- Opioids
- Parkinson's drugs
- Remember to ask about any recent use of medications which has stopped – medication withdrawal can lead to confusion

Family history
- Any hereditary neurological conditions, e.g. Huntington's
- Family history of stroke and cardiovascular disease

Social history
- Who patient lives with
- Social support network
- Alcohol and drug use

OSCE Key Learning Points

✔ It is essential to gain a collaborative history

 Common misinterpretations and pitfalls

It is easy to assume that because a patient has a diagnosis of dementia that their current level of confusion is normal for them. However, acute on chronic confusion is an important presenting complaint and it is therefore important to establish a patient's baseline state.

12 Constipation

Definition: Infrequent or difficult passage of abnormally hard/firm faeces.

Differentials

- *Medical*: diet, lifestyle, irritable bowel syndrome, hypercalcaemia, hypothyroidism, drugs (opiates, tricyclic antidepressants)
- *Surgical*: diverticular disease, anal fissure, carcinoma of the colon/rectum/anus, pelvic masses

History

Presenting complaint
- How many days since last bowel movement
- Normal frequency of stool
- Length of time affected by constipation
- Normal consistency of stool
- Consistency of stool now
  - Any associated pain with defecation
  - Any suggestion of overflow diarrhoea
- Any blood or mucus PR
- Associated symptoms
  - Abdominal pain
  - Bloating
  - Nausea/vomiting
  - Loss of appetite

Medical Student Survival Skills: History Taking and Communication Skills, First Edition.
Philip Jevon and Steve Odogwu.
© 2020 John Wiley & Sons Ltd. Published 2020 by John Wiley & Sons Ltd.
Companion website: www.wiley.com/go/jevon/medicalstudent

- Systems review
  - Any suggestion of urinary obstruction/difficulty
  - Muscular aches and pains
  - Recent weight loss/weight gain
  - Night sweats
  - Fatigue

Past medical and surgical history
- Hypothyroidism
- Chronic pain
  - Arthritis
  - Recent surgery/injuries
- Previous abdominal surgery
- Current or previous malignancies

Drug history
- Opiate use
- Laxative use
- Calcium supplements

Social history
- Smoker
- Diet
- Amount of fluid intake?
- Reduced fibre intake?
- Regular exercise

OSCE Key Learning Points

✔ Remember to ask about red flag symptoms – recent change in bowel habit, weight loss, mucus/altered blood PR

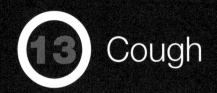 Cough

Definition: Forced expiration of air from lungs against an initially closed glottis.

Differentials

- *Common*: upper respiratory tract infection (URTI), pneumonia, gastro-oesophageal reflux disease (GORD), asthma, chronic obstructive pulmonary disease (COPD), pulmonary malignancy, drugs
- *Rare*: parenchymal lung disease, bronchiectasis, tuberculosis

History

History of presenting complaint
- Duration and frequency of symptoms – acute or chronic (>3 weeks)
- Description of cough
- Exacerbating factors
- Any sputum production
- Colour and quantity of sputum – haemoptysis, infective
- Associated pain: use SOCRATES template (see Chapter 8)
- Associated symptoms: shortness of breath, weight loss, coryzal symptoms, reflux

Past medical and surgical history
- Asthma, COPD, bronchiectasis, GORD
- Recent flu-like illness
- Any other illnesses

Medical Student Survival Skills: History Taking and Communication Skills, First Edition.
Philip Jevon and Steve Odogwu.
© 2020 John Wiley & Sons Ltd. Published 2020 by John Wiley & Sons Ltd.
Companion website: www.wiley.com/go/jevon/medicalstudent

Medications and allergies
- Current medications: angiotensin converting enzyme inhibitors (ACEIs), beta-blockers, inhalers
- Allergies

Family history
- Any family members with similar symptoms
- Any illnesses that run in the family

Social history
- Who patient lives with and type of accommodation
- Occupation (e.g. asbestos exposure or working with birds)
- Smoking and alcohol

OSCE Key Learning Points

✔ A description of the sputum can give you clues to the diagnosis

 NB Any history of weight loss or haemoptysis in a smoker should be rapidly investigated.

 Common misinterpretations and pitfalls

Most coughs are associated with viral URTIs but watch out for red flag symptoms.

(14) Deliberate self-harm

Definition: Deliberate self-harm (DSH) is a non-fatal act of self-injury and/or self-poisoning. Suicidal intent may or may not be present in varying degrees.

History

 NB History taking should be done sensitively, respectfully, and in an appropriately private environment. The offer of preferred gender clinician should be made if possible.

The history should focus on assessing the full extent of the injury/poisoning, the motivation behind it, and the risk of further DSH.

History of presenting complaint
- *Self-poisoning*
  - What was taken
  - How many tablets
  - What time
  - All at once or staggered
  - With alcohol
- *Self-harm*
  - What instrument was used – is it clean
  - What time
- *Points important to both*
  - What was the trigger that lead to the act – e.g. bereavement, loss of job
  - What was the intention of the act – ask specifically the intention to end their life

Medical Student Survival Skills: History Taking and Communication Skills, First Edition.
Philip Jevon and Steve Odogwu.
© 2020 John Wiley & Sons Ltd. Published 2020 by John Wiley & Sons Ltd.
Companion website: www.wiley.com/go/jevon/medicalstudent

37

- If yes – are they glad now that the act was not successful?
- Did they seek medical help themselves or were they forced to come
- Where did the act take place – in a place of privacy or a place where they were likely to be found
- Was there a suicide note left? Did the patient make a will recently?

Past medical and surgical history
- Psychiatric history
- Previous acts of DSH
- Chronic /terminal illnesses

Medications and allergies
- Ask about all prescription medications that the patient has access to
- Allergies

Family history
- Family history of psychiatric disorders

OSCE Key Learning Points

✔ The aim of the history is to assess suicidal risk and intent

✔ The SAD PERSONS score is a screening tool used to assess suicide risk after an act of deliberate self-harm. People scoring 5+ are deemed higher risk and must be referred to psychiatric services. Patients score points on the following criteria:

S	Sex – male gender = 1 point
A	Age: < 19 to > 45 = 1 point
D	Depression/hopelessness = 2 points
P	Previous attempts/psychiatric care = 1 point
E	Excessive alcohol use = 1 point
R	Rational thinking loss/organic brain disease = 2 points
S	Single widowed or divorced = 1 point
O	Organised/serious attempt = 2 points
N	No social support = 1 point
S	Stated future intent = 2 points

Social history

- Social support network
- Occupation
- Alcohol and drug use

 NB In the year following an act of self-harm 1–2% of patients will go on to complete suicide.

 Common misinterpretations and pitfalls

Not all acts of deliberate self-harm are genuine suicide attempts. However, it is very important to risk assess *all* acts of self-harm thoroughly.

(15) Diarrhoea

> **Definition:** Three or more loose or liquid bowel movements per day.

Differentials

- *Common*: gastroenteritis (viral and bacterial), inflammatory bowel disease, constipation (with overflow), bowel cancer, irritable bowel syndrome
- *Rare*: coeliac disease, iatrogenic (e.g. medications), parasitic

History

 NB Infection control measures.

History of presenting complaint
- Ascertain that stool is not formed or is liquid
- When it started
- Normal frequency of bowel motion
- Frequency
- Quantity
- Associated local pain
- Tenesmus
- Stool: colour, tarry (melaena), any blood or mucus
- Difficulty in flushing the stool
- Abdominal pain: aggravating or relieving factors
- Relation to foods like bread, cakes, oats, etc.
- Any weight loss or fever

Medical Student Survival Skills: History Taking and Communication Skills, First Edition.
Philip Jevon and Steve Odogwu.
© 2020 John Wiley & Sons Ltd. Published 2020 by John Wiley & Sons Ltd.
Companion website: www.wiley.com/go/jevon/medicalstudent

Past medical and surgical history
- Constipation or diarrhoea
- Diabetes mellitus, inflammatory bowel disease, any other illnesses
- Any previous surgery – especially gynaecological or abdominal

Medications and allergies
- Current medications
- Laxative use
- Recent antibiotics
- Allergies

Social history
- Who patient lives with: do other household members have symptoms?
- Smoking and alcohol
- Recent foreign travel
- Change in diet

OSCE Key Learning Points

✔ In particular, remember to ask about weight loss and recent travel

 NB Any change in bowel habit, especially in the elderly, should be fully investigated.

 Common misinterpretations and pitfalls

Establish early the stool consistency – some patients will report 'diarrhoea' after a couple of more soft-type stools.

16 Dizziness and vertigo

> **Definition:**
> - *Dizziness* is a term used by patients to describe many different sensations, including being off balance, light-headedness, and vertigo.
> - *Vertigo* is an illusion of movement, often rotatory, of the patient, or his surroundings.

Differentials of Vertigo

- *Common*: benign paroxysmal positional vertigo (BPPV), Meniere's disease, labyrinthitis, vestibular neuronitis, brainstem stroke/transient ischaemic attack (TIA), alcohol intoxication, multiple sclerosis (MS), motion sickness, ototoxic drugs, space occupying lesion
- *Rare*: migraine, acoustic neuroma

History

 NB Find out exactly what the patient means by the term dizziness.

History of presenting complaint
- Ascertain the exact description of patient sensation
- Onset – sudden or gradual
- Progression of symptoms
- Duration – how long do spells last

Medical Student Survival Skills: History Taking and Communication Skills, First Edition.
Philip Jevon and Steve Odogwu.
© 2020 John Wiley & Sons Ltd. Published 2020 by John Wiley & Sons Ltd.
Companion website: www.wiley.com/go/jevon/medicalstudent

- Triggers of symptoms – positional (head or postural)
- Any associated symptoms – loss of consciousness, nausea/vomiting, difficulty standing, hearing loss, tinnitus
- History of falls or traumas
- Other neurological symptoms or visual disturbance
- Weight loss or change in behaviour

Past medical and surgical history
- Previous neurological history: central nervous systsem (CNS) malignancy, MS, migraine, epilepsy
- Previous cerebrovascular accident (CVA), diabetes mellitus, postural hypotension
- History of any malignancy
- Any previous ear, nose, and throat surgery

Medications and allergies
- Current medications
- Antihypertensive medications
- Aminoglycosides
- Allergies

Social history
- Alcohol intake
- Occupation

Family history
- Family history of CVA, cancers (including CNS malignancy) or migraine

OSCE Key Learning Points

✔ In particular, remember to ask about triggers and duration of dizzy spells
✔ On examination look for change of symptoms with position, ability to walk, focal neurology, and cerebellar signs (using the DANISH approach: **d**ysdiadochokinesia, **a**taxia, **n**ystagmus, **i**ntention tremor, **s**lurred speech, and **h**ypotonia)

NB Worrying features include associated focal neurology.

 Common misinterpretations and pitfalls

Dizziness is a non-specific term. It is very important to ascertain what sensation the patient is exactly experiencing when feeling dizzy.

17 Dyspepsia

Definition: Pain or discomfort in the epigastrium/upper abdomen.

Differentials

- *Common*: gastro-oesophageal reflux disease (GORD), *Helicobacter pylori*, alcohol, hiatus hernias, peptic ulcers, drugs, functional dyspepsia (no clear cause found)
- *Rare*: malignancy

History

History of presenting complaint
- Ask the patient to describe the actual sensation they experience
- When it started
- Constant dyspepsia, or comes and goes
- Any epigastric pain
- Associated symptoms – nausea, vomiting, belching, bloating, dysphagia, bowel symptoms – stool, flatus, melaena
- Exacerbating and relieving factors
- Dyspepsia triggered by any particular foods/drink – spicy foods, coffee, alcohol
- Symptoms of anaemia – shortness of breath (SOB), lethargy, fatigue
- Red flag symptoms – weight loss, loss of appetite, night sweats, lymphadenopathy

Past medical history
- Inflammatory bowel disease
- Irritable bowel syndrome

Medical Student Survival Skills: History Taking and Communication Skills, First Edition.
Philip Jevon and Steve Odogwu.
© 2020 John Wiley & Sons Ltd. Published 2020 by John Wiley & Sons Ltd.
Companion website: www.wiley.com/go/jevon/medicalstudent

- Known GORD or hiatus hernia
- Any previous abdominal surgery

Medications and allergies
Ask specifically about drugs that can irritate the lining of the stomach and increase acid reflux:

- Aspirin/anticoagulants, non-steroidal anti-inflammatory drugs (NSAIDs)
- Calcium channel blockers
- Nitrates
- Anticholinergics – these will decrease gut motility

Family history
- Bowel cancer or other malabsorptive disorders

Social history
- Smoking – this is a risk factor for both gastric and oesophageal cancers
- Alcohol – can cause peptic ulcers
- Effect of symptoms on daily life

OSCE Key Learning Points

✔ In particular, when taking a medication history do not forget to specifically ask about over the counter (OTC) medications – there are plenty of patients who take OTC NSAIDs and do not disclose this until you specifically ask!

 Common misinterpretations and pitfalls

Cardiac disease can present as dyspepsia/upper gastrointestinal symptoms. Always enquire about palpitations, SOB, nausea, and sweating – this can catch you out!

(18) Dysphagia

Definition: Difficulty in swallowing.

Differentials

Mechanical block	Motility disorders	Others
Malignant stricture:	Achalasia	Oesophagitis
Oesophageal, gastric, or pharyngeal cancer	Systemic sclerosis	
Benign strictures:	Myasthenia gravis	
Oesophageal web or ring	Bulbar palsy	
Peptic stricture	Oesophageal spasm	
Extrinsic pressure:		
Lung cancer, retrosternal goitre, aortic aneurysm		
Pharyngeal pouch		

History

 NB Dysphagia always needs to be investigated urgently to exclude malignancy unless it is of short duration or associated with a sore throat.

History of presenting complaint
- When did it start – acute versus chronic
- Was it difficult to swallow solids and liquids from the start – if the answer is yes, then it is a motility disorder. If the answer is no, it was solids initially then liquids, then it is a stricture (benign or malignant)
- Is it painful to swallow (this is called odynophagia) – if yes, suspect cancer
- Is the difficulty in swallowing intermittent or constant – if intermittent, think of oesophageal spasm. If constant and getting worse, suspect cancer

Medical Student Survival Skills: History Taking and Communication Skills, First Edition.
Philip Jevon and Steve Odogwu.
© 2020 John Wiley & Sons Ltd. Published 2020 by John Wiley & Sons Ltd.
Companion website: www.wiley.com/go/jevon/medicalstudent

- Is it difficult to make the swallowing movement – if yes, think of neurological causes like bulbar palsy
- Does your neck bulge or gurgle on drinking – if the answer is yes, think of pharyngeal pouch
- Any weight loss

Past medical and surgical history
- Gastro-oesophageal reflux disease
- Previous upper gastrointestinal (GI) surgery (may lead to strictures)
- Previous stroke/transient ischaemic attack (TIA)
- Known head and neck or upper GI malignancy

Medications and allergies
- Current medications
- Allergies

Social history
- History of smoking
- Alcohol excess

OSCE Key Learning Points

✔ Your main aim during history taking is to establish whether the dysphagia is due to a mechanical cause or a motility disorder

 NB If the patient can swallow liquids but struggles with solids, then it is a mechanical block.

 Common misinterpretations and pitfalls

Make sure you know the difference between dysphagia (difficulty in swallowing) and odynophagia (pain on swallowing).

⓳ Dysphasia

Definition:
- *Dysphasia* is an acquired deficit in the comprehension or production of language.
- *Receptive dysphasia* (Wernicke's) is fluent speech, but comprehension is impaired.
- *Expressive dysphasia* (Broca's) is non-fluent speech, but comprehension is intact.

Differentials

- *Common*: cerebrovascular event (stroke/transient ischaemic attack [TIA]), head trauma, space occupying lesion, dementia

History

NB Optimise communication abilities; may need collateral history.

History of presenting complaint
- Onset and duration of dysphasia
- Progression of symptoms
- Associated neurological symptoms, such as weakness or numbness
- History of trauma/head injury
- History of seizures, memory loss or change in personality
- Previous episodes
- Any weight loss

Medical Student Survival Skills: History Taking and Communication Skills, First Edition.
Philip Jevon and Steve Odogwu.
© 2020 John Wiley & Sons Ltd. Published 2020 by John Wiley & Sons Ltd.
Companion website: www.wiley.com/go/jevon/medicalstudent

51

Past medical history
- Previous neurology, intracranial mass, psychiatric disorder, dementia
- Cardiovascular disease, hypertension, diastolic murmur, previous myocardial infarction, stroke, or TIA
- Bleeding disorder – thrombophilia, vasculitis
- Any malignancy

Medications and allergies
- Current medications
- Anticoagulation
- Sedatives and antipsychotics
- Allergies

Social history
- Who patient lives with and daily living activities
- Alcohol intake
- Smoking

OSCE Key Learning Points

✔ In particular, do not forget to ask about onset and progression of symptoms, as patient might be suitable for thrombolysis if presenting within the time window

 NB National Institute for Health and Care Excellence guidelines recommend thrombolysis in patients presenting with ischaemic stroke within 4.5 hours from the onset of symptoms.

 Common misinterpretations and pitfalls

Involve witnesses and establish early on the onset and duration of symptoms as this determines the subsequent management plans.

20 Dysuria

> **Definition:** Pain on urinating.

Differentials

- *Women*: urethritis, gynaecological causes, pyelonephritis, urinary tract infections (UTIs), sexually transmitted infections (STIs)
- *Men*:
  - *<50 years of age: STIs, urolithiasis*
  - *>50 years of age: UTIs, pyelonep*hritis, benign prostatic hyperplasia (BPH)

History

History of presenting complaint
- Onset, duration, and nature of symptoms
- Urinary frequency
- Suprapubic pain, loin to groin pain (SOCRATES approach, see Chapter 8)
- Pyrexia, rigors
- Catheter in situ
- Detailed sexual history
- Men: bladder outflow obstruction – straining to void, poor stream, terminal dribbling
- Women: last menstrual period – rule out pregnancy
- Red flag symptoms: weight loss, haematuria

Past medical and surgical history
- Previous UTIs, known renal disease
- Malignancy

Medical Student Survival Skills: History Taking and Communication Skills, First Edition.
Philip Jevon and Steve Odogwu.
© 2020 John Wiley & Sons Ltd. Published 2020 by John Wiley & Sons Ltd.
Companion website: www.wiley.com/go/jevon/medicalstudent

- Diabetes, immunocompromised
- Any abdominal or urological surgery

Medications and allergies
- Allergies
- Current medications
- Anticholinergics

Family history
- Any medical conditions that run in the family
- Family history of malignancy

Social history
- Who patient lives with, type of housing
- Occupation; exposure to chemicals
- Smoking and alcohol
- Recent foreign travel

OSCE Key Learning Points

✔ Duration and nature of symptoms will help to differentiate between diagnoses

 NB Any red flag symptoms such as haematuria should be investigated.

 Common misinterpretations and pitfalls

Forgetting to take a sexual history where indicated.

21 Otalgia – ear ache

Definition:
- *Primary otalgia* is pain originating from the ear.
- *Referred otalgia* is pain originating from outside the ear but perceived as from the ear.

Differentials

- *External ear*: otitis externa, foreign body, perichondritis, impacted wax, trauma, Ramsay Hunt syndrome, malignant otitis externa, neoplasm
- *Internal ear*: otitis media, tympanic membrane perforation (barotrauma), mastoiditis, neoplasm
- *Referred*: tonsillitis, dental infections, nasopharyngeal carcinoma, tonsillar carcinoma, laryngeal carcinoma, temporomandibular joint dysfunction

History

History of presenting complaint
- Onset, site, and duration of pain
- Progression and severity of the pain, e.g. scoring
- Exacerbating and relieving factors
- Any preceding illness or symptoms, e.g. viral illness
- Any discharge from the ears – colour, smell
- Any hearing loss or tinnitus (ringing)
- Any associated vertigo symptoms
- History of trauma or foreign body in ear, e.g. cotton buds
- Recent deep water diving or air travel
- Any weight loss or fever

Medical Student Survival Skills: History Taking and Communication Skills, First Edition.
Philip Jevon and Steve Odogwu.
© 2020 John Wiley & Sons Ltd. Published 2020 by John Wiley & Sons Ltd.
Companion website: www.wiley.com/go/jevon/medicalstudent

- Any dysphagia, odynophagia, or hoarseness of voice
- Any weight loss, fever

Past medical and surgical history
- Diabetes, immunosuppression, human immunodeficiency virus (HIV)
- Any previous ear problems or surgery
- Any dental problems

Medications and allergies
- Current medications – important to look out for cytotoxic drugs and steroids
- Allergies

Family history
- Any family members with similar symptoms
- Any illnesses that run in the family

Social history
- Who patient lives with
- Occupation
- Smoking and alcohol
- Recent foreign travel

OSCE Key Learning Points

✔ In particular, remember to ask about discharge, tinnitus, and vertigo

NB
- A discharging, painful ear in diabetic patients or immunosuppressed patients should raise the possibility of malignant otitis externa
- Always be prepared to ask about referred sources of otalgia – a thorough examination will help identify these

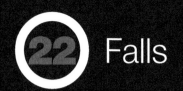

22 Falls

Definition: An event that results in a person coming to rest inadvertently on the ground or floor or other lower level.

Differentials

- *Simple*: trip, knocked down, poor footwear
- *Neurological*: seizure, impaired vision, stroke, impaired sensation in feet, cerebellar problems, balance loss
- *Cardiovascular*: postural hypotension, myocardial infarction, arrhythmia
- *Respiratory*: pulmonary embolus, pneumothorax
- *Vascular*: ruptured aortic aneurysm, subarachnoid haemorrhage
- *Infection*: any, especially in the elderly

 Common misinterpretations and pitfalls

Often the term 'fall' incorrectly encompasses syncope, collapse, or loss of consciousness. Patients can be labelled as having fallen, yet a more sinister symptom has resulted in the fall – e.g. seizure or chest pain. It is important to draw out discriminating points in the history.

Medical Student Survival Skills: History Taking and Communication Skills, First Edition.
Philip Jevon and Steve Odogwu.
© 2020 John Wiley & Sons Ltd. Published 2020 by John Wiley & Sons Ltd.
Companion website: www.wiley.com/go/jevon/medicalstudent

57

History

History of presenting complaint

OSCE Key Learning Tip

✔ Split your questions into what happened before, during, and after the fall. That way you will not miss any important pieces of information. This technique works well with most symptoms – e.g. chest pain (before pain: was walking; during pain: nausea, shortness of breath; after pain: sat down and took glyceryl trinitrate, which helped)

- What happened before the 'fall'
  - Did they trip; were they walking about or had just stood up
  - Loss of consciousness, lightheaded, dizzy, severe headache
  - Chest pain, palpitation, shortness of breath
  - Important for the elderly: what footwear, use of recommended aids
- What happened during the fall
  - What did they fall onto (hands, face, hip, floor, radiator, down steps)
  - What injuries did they sustain – ask specifically about head injury
  - Did they appear to fit – any eye witnesses
- What happened after the fall
  - Could they get up afterwards

Past medical and surgical history
- Any previous falls or fractures as a result of fall
- Medical problems increasing risk of falls in elderly include joint disease, dementia, and sensory impairment (blind/deaf). Also consider any childhood problems that could influence mobility – e.g. polio

Medications and allergies
- Especially antihypertensives, sedatives, and heart rate slowing medications
- Any known allergies

Family history
- Any illnesses that run in the family

Social history
- For the elderly:
  - Where do they live – house, any stairs, nursing home
  - Who do they live with – do they have any care from family or carers
  - Do they have any aids to walk with usually
- Occupation – especially important if patient has lost consciousness or cause is unclear, as this may prevent them returning to work until the cause is established
- Smoking and alcohol

 NB For elderly patients check what aids they usually use for walking, foot wear, and glasses in use at the time of the fall. Are they on any medications that could influence their balance or cognition? Do they have any neurological, cardiovascular, cognitive, or joint diseases that could contribute to a fall?

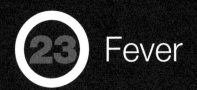
Fever

Definition: Body temperature raised above 37 °C (also called pyrexia).

Differentials

- *Common*: viral infections, bacterial infections, connective tissue disorders, malignancy
- *Rare*: drugs (e.g. phenytoin)

 NB Pyrexia of unknown origin (PUO) is fever for more than 3 weeks with no obvious cause despite adequate investigation.

 Common misinterpretations and pitfalls

Remember that fever/pyrexia only refers to a raised temperature (not any associated features) and is not only caused by infection.

History

History of presenting complaint
- Duration
- Shivering or rigors
- Headache
- Nausea or vomiting
- Constipation or diarrhoea
- Rashes

Medical Student Survival Skills: History Taking and Communication Skills, First Edition.
Philip Jevon and Steve Odogwu.
© 2020 John Wiley & Sons Ltd. Published 2020 by John Wiley & Sons Ltd.
Companion website: www.wiley.com/go/jevon/medicalstudent

- Joint pain or inflammation
- Lumps or masses (e.g. lympadenopathy)
- Respiratory symptoms (e.g. cough)
- Urinary symptoms (e.g. dysuria)
- Delirium or convulsions

 NB Delirium and convulsions may occur above 40.5 °C, particularly in young children.

Past medical and surgical history
- Recurrent infections
- Previous illnesses
- Any previous surgery or accidents

 NB Consider deep vein thrombosis as a cause of fever in a postoperative patient.

Medications and allergies
- Current medications
- Immunosuppressants
- Immunisations
- Allergies

Family history
- Any illnesses that run in the family

Social history
- Recent foreign travel
- Sexual history
- Contact with infected people
- Animal contact
- Smoking and alcohol
- IV drug use

OSCE Key Learning Points

✔ A septic screen involves getting bloods (full blood count, urea and electrolytes, C-reactive protein), a chest X-ray, and taking cultures from every possible site (e.g. blood, urine, stool, sputum, cerebrospinal fluid)

(24) Haematemesis

> **Definition:** The presence of blood in vomit.

Differentials

- *Common*: peptic ulcers, Mallory–Weiss tear, oesophageal varices, gastritis/gastric erosions, drugs (non-steroidal anti-inflammatory drugs [NSAIDs], aspirin, steroids, thrombolytics, anticoagulants), oesophagitis, duodenitis, malignancy, no obvious cause
- *Rare*: bleeding disorders, portal hypertensive gastropathy, aorto-enteric fistula, angiodysplasia, haemobilia, Meckel's diverticulum, Peutz–Jeghers syndrome, Osler–Weber–Rendu syndrome

History

 NB Take a brief history and examine the patient to assess severity.

History of presenting complaint
- When it first started – acute or chronic
- Any previous gastrointestinal (GI) bleeds, dyspepsia
- What colour is the blood (dark red-brown 'coffee grounds' is old or small-volume stomach bleeding; dark red may be venous from the oesophagus; bright red is arterial and often from a major gastric or duodenal artery)
- What volume over what period? Helps you assess severity
- Did the blood appear with the initial vomits or after a period of prolonged vomiting (suggests oesophageal traumatic cause)
- Any chest or abdominal pain

Medical Student Survival Skills: History Taking and Communication Skills, First Edition.
Philip Jevon and Steve Odogwu.
© 2020 John Wiley & Sons Ltd. Published 2020 by John Wiley & Sons Ltd.
Companion website: www.wiley.com/go/jevon/medicalstudent

- Ask about melaena (black, tar-like, foul-smelling motions, indicating upper gastrointestinal bleeding)
- Any weight loss (suggesting possible malignancy)
- Ask about dysphagia (difficulty swallowing), suggesting possible malignancy

Past medical history
- Known gastro-oesophageal reflux disease or peptic ulcers
- Known liver disease or oesophageal varices
- Any serious co-morbidities like cardiovascular, respiratory, hepatic, or renal disease (worse prognosis)
- Known malignancy

Medications and allergies
- Current medications especially NSAIDs, aspirin, clopidogrel, steroids, anticoagulants
- Are they on proton pump inhibitors (PPIs), e.g. omeprazole, lansoprazole
- Allergies

Social history
- History of alcohol excess
- Smoking history

OSCE Key Learning Points

✔ A patient coming to hospital with any form of bleeding should be stabilised first using ABCDE along with IV access and group and save or cross match before any investigation

 Common misinterpretations and pitfalls

Make sure it is haematemesis and not haemoptysis (coughing blood).

25 Haematuria

Definition: Presence of blood in the urine, which may be:
- Macroscopic – visible to the naked eye
- Microscopic – detected by either dipstick testing or by analysis under a microscope

Differentials

- *Renal causes*: renal cancer, glomerulonephritis, infection, polycystic kidney, pyelonephritis, calculi
- *Extrarenal causes*: bladder/prostate/urethral cancer, cystitis/prostatitis/urethritis, calculi, trauma (catheters very common!), disorders of coagulation/anticoagulants

These are merely some of the most common causes, the actual list is extensive!

History

 NB Infection control measures.

History of presenting complaint
- Location – blood may actually originate from the vagina or rectum
- Timing – early stream suggests urethra or prostate, mid-stream suggests bladder, terminal bleeding suggests kidney
- Amount/presence of clots

Medical Student Survival Skills: History Taking and Communication Skills, First Edition.
Philip Jevon and Steve Odogwu.
© 2020 John Wiley & Sons Ltd. Published 2020 by John Wiley & Sons Ltd.
Companion website: www.wiley.com/go/jevon/medicalstudent

67

- Associated symptoms – dysuria, renal colic, irritative symptoms (frequency, nocturia, urgency – suggests stones, urinary tract infection, cancer), constitutional symptoms
- Recent trauma or vigorous exercise (rhabdomyolysis)
- Diet – beetroot turns urine red!

Past medical and surgical history
- Renal stones
- Urinary tract infections
- Cancer
- Bleeding disorders
- Any previous urinary tract surgery

Medications and allergies
- Rifampacin/nitrofurantoin – turn urine red
- Anticoagulants/antiplatelets
- Any known allergies

Social history
- Smoking and alcohol
- Recent foreign travel
- Occupation/chemical exposure
- First degree relatives with renal tract disease

OSCE Key Learning Points

✔ Painless haematuria is more worrying – cancer is the most likely cause

 NB Macroscopic haematuria should always be fully investigated, as should microscopic haematuria in the over 50s.

 Common misinterpretations and pitfalls

Timing and associated symptoms are key to making the right diagnosis.

(26) Haemoptysis

Definition: Spitting or coughing up of blood or blood-streaked mucus from the respiratory tract.

Differentials

- *Common*: tuberculosis (TB), malignancy, pulmonary embolism, bronchiectasis, pneumonia
- *Rare*: vasculitis (Granulomatosis with polyangiitis (GPA) formerly known as Wegener's granulomatosis), Goodpasture's syndrome, lung abscess

History

History of presenting complaint
- Onset: sudden, gradual, duration, number of episodes, daily/intermittent
- Obtain description of haemoptysis: frank blood, blood-stained, volume, colour pink, and frothy/bright red/rusty
- Associations: cough, shortness of breath, sputum, chest pain, leg swelling (deep vein thrombosis [DVT])
- Precipitating factors: throat/chest infection, risk factors for DVT (immobilisation), contact with anyone with TB, trauma, foreign body inhalation
- Any bleeding elsewhere: haematuria, epistaxis
- Any weight loss, night sweats

Past medical and surgical history
- Previous history of TB or TB treatment
- History of coagulation disorders/vasculitis
- Any other illnesses, including childhood infections

Medical Student Survival Skills: History Taking and Communication Skills, First Edition.
Philip Jevon and Steve Odogwu.
© 2020 John Wiley & Sons Ltd. Published 2020 by John Wiley & Sons Ltd.
Companion website: www.wiley.com/go/jevon/medicalstudent

Medications and allergies
- Current medications; anticoagulants
- Allergies

Family history
- Any family members with similar symptoms
- Any illnesses that run in the family; malignancy, coagulopathies

Social history
- Smoking – how much and for how long, current/ex-smoker
- Travel history
- Occupation (exposures, e.g. asbestos)
- Mobility; how far can you normally walk without stopping, mobility aids

OSCE Key Learning Points

✔ In particular, remember to ask about weight loss, recent travel, and smoking

 NB Red flags include weight loss, night sweats, and smoking, and will require further investigation.

 Common misinterpretations and pitfalls

Establish whether it is true haemoptysis – differentiate between epistaxis and haematemesis.

27 Headache

Definition: Pain anywhere in the region of the head.

Differentials

- *Common*: migraine, tension-type headache
- *Rare*: subarachnoid haemorrhage (SAH), meningitis, encephalitis, raised intracranial pressure (ICP), giant cell arteritis, cluster headache

History

History of presenting complaint
- Site – where is the pain, unilateral/bilateral
- Onset; sudden (seconds, minutes), gradual (hours, days). How often do you get the headaches (e.g. frequent)
- Character; stabbing, aching; did it feel like you were 'Hit over the back your head'?
- Radiation
- Associated symptoms:
  - Fever, neck stiffness, photophobia, drowsiness, rash
  - Loss of consciousness (LOC), vomiting
  - Aura, limb weakness
  - Scalp tenderness, jaw pain, loss of vision
  - Seizure
  - Drowsy, change in personality
- Timing – intermittent/constant, how long do they last, worse at any particular time of day
- Exacerbating – worse on lying down/coughing/straining

Medical Student Survival Skills: History Taking and Communication Skills, First Edition.
Philip Jevon and Steve Odogwu.
© 2020 John Wiley & Sons Ltd. Published 2020 by John Wiley & Sons Ltd.
Companion website: www.wiley.com/go/jevon/medicalstudent

- Relieving – better when resting; better with medication
- Severity – does it prevent you from doing anything, e.g. work. Score the pain out of 10
- Under any stress at work/home

Past medical and surgical history
- Migraines, glaucoma
- Any other illnesses
- Any previous surgery/recent lumbar puncture

Medications and allergies
- Current medications; use of: glyceryl nitrate, combined oral contraceptive pill (COCP), codeine
- Allergies

Social history
- Any family members with similar symptoms
- Any sudden deaths in the family
- Any illnesses that run in the family
- Diet – cheese, chocolate, red wine
- Recent foreign travel
- Smoking and alcohol
- Occupation

OSCE Key Learning Points

✔ In particular, do not forget to ask about:
- Whether it felt like being hit over the back of the head
- LOC, vomiting
- Neck stiffness, photophobia

NB Headaches can be life-threatening! So *always* exclude meningitis and SAH in anyone who has presented with a headache. Migraines can present similarly to SAH. If in doubt about the diagnosis, always check with a senior.

28 Hoarseness

Definition: Abnormality in voice to a deeper, rougher, and harsher sound quality.

Differentials

- *Inflammatory*: acute laryngitis, tuberculosis, laryngopharyngeal reflux disease
- *Benign laryngeal condition*: voice overuse, laryngeal cord haemorrhage, benign lesion, e.g. polyp, papilloma, cysts
- *Malignant lesions*: laryngeal cancer, thyroid cancer, mediastinal tumours
- *Neurological*: recurrent laryngeal nerve palsy (unilateral), stroke, Parkinson's disease, myasthenia gravis
- *Endocrine*: hypothyroidism, acromegaly

History

History of presenting complaint
- Onset and duration of symptoms
- Any precipitating factor for onset, e.g. viral illness, aspiration, change in voice use
- Progression of symptom
- Any lumps felt in neck
- Associated symptoms: dysphagia, lump sensation in throat, haemoptysis, otalgia, difficulty in breathing, acid taste in mouth, heartburn
- Recent trauma or surgery to neck or chest
- Smoking history
- Any weight loss, fevers

Medical Student Survival Skills: History Taking and Communication Skills, First Edition.
Philip Jevon and Steve Odogwu.
© 2020 John Wiley & Sons Ltd. Published 2020 by John Wiley & Sons Ltd.
Companion website: www.wiley.com/go/jevon/medicalstudent

Past medical and surgical history
- Previous intubation
- Any thyroid or cardiothoracic surgery
- Neurological or endocrinology history

Medications and allergies
- Current medications
- Allergies

Family history
- Any illnesses that run in the family

Social history
- Who patient lives with
- Occupation very important, e.g. singer, teacher
- Smoking history

OSCE Key Learning Points

✔ Always consider laryngeal cancer in those with a significant smoking history

 NB Remember the left recurrent laryngeal originates from the vagus nerve in the thorax and winds around the arch of aorta before ascending to the larynx.

 NB Hoarseness may be a result of systemic disease.

29 Jaundice

Definition: Yellow skin or sclera, which is due to high plasma bilirubin.

 NB Jaundice may be a symptom reported by the patient or a physical sign noticed on physical examination. Plasma levels usually need to be over 35 μmol l^{-1} for high bilirubin levels to become clinically apparent as jaundice.

Differentials

- *Pre-hepatic*: haemolysis (hereditary or acquired haemolytic anaemia, septicaemic haemolysis, malaria), Gilbert's syndrome, Crigler–Najjar syndrome
- *Hepatic*: hepatitis (infective, drug-induced, alcoholic), glandular fever, cirrhosis, liver metastases/abscess, haemochromatosis, Wilson's disease, alpha-1 antitrypsin deficiency, Budd–Chiari syndrome
- *Post-hepatic*: obstructive (gallstones, head of pancreas cancer, cholangiocarcinoma, sclerosing cholangitis, primary biliary cirrhosis)

History

 NB Infection control measures with bodily fluids.

History of presenting complaint
- Onset and duration
- Has the jaundice worsened/stayed the same or improved

Medical Student Survival Skills: History Taking and Communication Skills, First Edition.
Philip Jevon and Steve Odogwu.
© 2020 John Wiley & Sons Ltd. Published 2020 by John Wiley & Sons Ltd.
Companion website: www.wiley.com/go/jevon/medicalstudent

- Associated symptoms:
  - Change in bowel habits, especially steatorrhoea
  - Pruritis
  - Dark urine
  - Fever/rigors
  - Bruising
  - Lethargy
  - Weight loss/change in clothes size
  - Nausea and vomiting
  - Abdominal pain
  - Regurgitation
  - Abdominal distension
  - In a young adult, history of dysarthria, dyskinesias, dystonias, ataxia, personality change, depression, parkinsonism, dementia (signs of Wilson's disease).

Past medical and surgical history
- History of hepatitis/alcoholic liver disease/autoimmune disease
- History of emphysema
- History of blood transfusions
- History of psychiatric problems or overdose
- Any other illnesses or any previous surgeries

Medications and allergies
- Current medications, especially: antimalarials, paracetamol, statins, sodium valproate, antibiotics, prochlorperazine
- Compliance with medications
- Allergy history

Family history
- Hereditary liver disease: Wilson's disease, haemochromatosis, alpha-1 antitrypsin deficiency, Gilbert's syndrome, Crigler–Najjar syndrome
- Any medical conditions running in the family

Social history
- Who patient lives with
- Current mobility and ability to do activities of daily living
- Current housing situation – bungalow/stairs
- Occupation history
- Smoking history

- Recent travel
- Alcohol history and IV drug use
- Sexual health
- Any body piercings/tattoos

OSCE Key Learning Points

✔ Consider malignancy in a patient with painless jaundice

 NB Pre-hepatic (unconjugated hyperbilirubinaemia): normal-coloured stools and urine; hepatic (conjugated and unconjugated hyperbilirubinaemia): normal-coloured stools with dark urine; post-hepatic (conjugated hyperbilirubinaemia): pale stools with dark urine.

Common misinterpretations and pitfalls

Patients may accidentally take a gradual overdose of paracetamol. If paracetamol is regularly taken, ask how often and at what dose. If patient is in hospital check the drug chart and their weight: If their weight is less than 50 kg, they should receive a lower dose (15 mg kg^{-1}).

(30) Joint pain

Definition: Arthralgia or joint pain is pain felt in any of the body's joints.

Differentials

- *Causes of joint pain include*: Osteoarthritis, rheumatoid arthritis, gout, pseudo-gout, septic arthritis, reactive arthritis, psoriatic arthritis, malignancy, osteomyelitis, systemic lupus erythematosus, inflammatory bowel disease, rheumatic fever

History

History of presenting complaint
- Joint pain – use SOCRATES approach (see Chapter 8)
  - Onset – acute versus chronic
  - Character – sharp and stabbing, boring/penetrating, shooting pain
  - Pattern of distribution
- Stiffness – relation to time of day, localised/generalised, relation to activity/rest
- Swelling – joints affected, distribution, speed of onset, constant/intermittent
- Deformity – acute/chronic development
- History of trauma
- Locking
- Weakness – localised/generalised
- Sensory disturbance – distribution
- Extra-articular features
  - Systemic – fever, night sweats, weight loss, lethargy
  - Skin – rashes, psoriasis, bruising

Medical Student Survival Skills: History Taking and Communication Skills, First Edition.
Philip Jevon and Steve Odogwu.
© 2020 John Wiley & Sons Ltd. Published 2020 by John Wiley & Sons Ltd.
Companion website: www.wiley.com/go/jevon/medicalstudent

- Eye – dry eyes, vision problems, pain
- Cardiorespiratory – shortness of breath, chest pain
- Gastrointestinal – abdominal pain, diarrhoea, constipation, PR bleeding
- Other: mouth/genital ulcers, change with sunlight, dysuria, sore throat

Past medical and surgical history
- Any other illnesses
- Previous joint pain
- Previous trauma
- Clotting abnormalities
- Psoriasis
- Previous surgery
- Joint surgery

Medications and allergies
- Allergies
- Current medications
- Particularly anticoagulants, steroids, thiazide diuretics

Family history
- Psoriasis
- Arthritis
- Autoimmune disease

Social history
- Occupation
- Effect on lifestyle, loss of function
- Dominant hand

OSCE Key Learning Points

✔ Remember to ask about extra-articular symptoms

 NB Septic arthritis is an emergency.

 Common misinterpretations and pitfalls

Referred pain, e.g. hip pathology presenting as knee pain.

31 Acute leg pain (ischaemic leg)

Definition: Acute limb ischaemia is defined as the sudden interruption of blood supply to a limb, usually secondary to a thrombus (85%) or an embolus (15%).

NB Thrombus formation usually occurs over a longer time period secondary to peripheral vascular disease. This is differentiated from chronic limb ischaemia, as the features usually present within a 2 week period.

Differentials

- *Common*: musculoskeletal pain, deep vein thrombosis (DVT), cellulitis, thrombophlebitis, sciatica, ruptured Baker's cyst
- *Life-threatening*: acute limb ischaemia, compartment syndrome, septic arthritis, sickle cell crisis, spinal cord compression

History

History of presenting complaint
- SOCRATES approach as in any pain history taking (see Chapter 8)
- Onset – sudden or chronic
- Loss in sensation/power
- Preceding trauma
- Any change in character of pain on raising leg. Does pain improve at night when hanging leg over side of bed (= critical ischaemia)
- Recent shortness of breath = DVT?

Medical Student Survival Skills: History Taking and Communication Skills, First Edition.
Philip Jevon and Steve Odogwu.
© 2020 John Wiley & Sons Ltd. Published 2020 by John Wiley & Sons Ltd.
Companion website: www.wiley.com/go/jevon/medicalstudent

81

- Change in temperature of limbs – 'perishing cold'
- Pain on weight bearing
- Colour change in leg on raising leg?
- Fever
- Swelling.
- Any new ulcers?
- Any hair loss? Any loss in muscle in legs?

Past medical and surgical history
- Recent surgery – DVT, previous grafts inserted
- Previous limb pain
- Do they have vasculopathy – diastolic murmur, myocardial infarction, cerebrovascular accident, DVT/pulmonary embolism,
- Recent plaster of Paris immobilisation = compartment syndrome risk
- Atrial fibrillation – source of 80% of all embolis resulting in acute limb ischaemia
- Malignancy – source of emboli, bone metastases
- Prosthetic limbs – risk of septic arthritis
- Thrombophilia
- Prosthetic heart valves as a source of emboli

Drug history
- On warfarin – is the international normalised ratio (INR) in a subtherapeutic range
- Immunosuppression (e.g. long-term steroids or chemotherapy) – at risk of septic arthritis
- Statins – rhabdomyolysis
- Beta-blockers are contraindicated in limb ischaemia
- Oestrogen therapy (e.g. oral contraceptive pill) a risk factor for DVTs

Social history
- Smoking history
- Exercise tolerance – in particular ask about claudication distance
- IV drug use – risk of thrombophlebitis
- Diet – is there high cholesterol

OSCE Key Learning Points

✔ Features suggestive of acute limb ischaemia:
- Rapidly worsening of symptoms such as pain
- 6 'P's = pain, pulseless, pallor (or mottling if severe), paralysis, parasthesia, perishingly cold
- Worsening exercise tolerance
- Relief in pain when hanging over side of bed

✔ Complete ischaemia leads to extensive necrosis if not dealt with within 6 hours of presentation. This is a *surgical emergency*

✔ Make sure to discuss primary and secondary prevention of cardio-vascular disease

NB Limb ischaemia is often a common cause of litigation, as delays in diagnosis can lead to unnecessary amputation and mortality. Commonly confused with sciatica, it becomes important to also conduct a thorough vascular examination. Omit to conduct Doppler investigation at your own peril!

32 Leg ulcer

Definition: Discontinuity or break in the skin of varying depths that fail to heal.

Differentials

- *Common*: arterial insufficiency (ischaemic), venous insufficiency, neuropathy, pressure sore
- *Rare*: skin cancers, skin infections

History

History of presenting complaint
- *Likely arterial background*:
  - Pain – constant versus on exercise
  - Pallor – particularly on elevation
  - Perishingly cold peripheries
  - Paraesthesia/paralysis
  - Nails – brittle and crumbly
  - Skin – hair loss, shiny, dry
  - Ulcer:
    - Site – bony prominences (pressure areas) on feet
    - Shape – regular, punched out, indolent
    - Base – deep, may be black, involving tendon/bone
- *Likely venous background:*
  - Varicose veins
  - Pain – worse on standing, relieved by walking
  - Blue/purple lower legs

Medical Student Survival Skills: History Taking and Communication Skills, First Edition.
Philip Jevon and Steve Odogwu.
© 2020 John Wiley & Sons Ltd. Published 2020 by John Wiley & Sons Ltd.
Companion website: www.wiley.com/go/jevon/medicalstudent

- Ankle swelling – improved in the morning
- Ulcer:
  - Site – medial/lateral malleoli
  - Shape – irregular
  - Base – shallow, pink, granulating
- *Likely diabetic neuropathy background*:
  - Sensory loss – no pain – trauma remains unnoticed
  - Motor loss – abnormal foot movement can lead to bony point exposure
  - Autonomic loss – dry, scaling, fissuring feet
  - Ulcer:
    - Ischaemic (arterial) component may be present
    - Site – weight bearing surfaces
    - Shape – regular
    - Base – variable depth, granulation
- *Likely pressure ulcer*:
  - Bed bound
  - Weakness – cannot change position
  - Ulcer
    - On pressure points (sacrum, coccyx, hips, heels)
    - Non-blanchable redness leads to tissue loss and exposed bone/ muscle

Past medical and surgical history
- Peripheral vascular disease
- Varicose veins/chronic venous insufficiency
- Diabetes (especially type II)
- Bedbound
- Hypertension
- Hypercholesterolaemia
- Obesity
- Previous vascular surgery (arterial or venous, on any part of the lower limb vascular tree)

Medications and allergies
- Current medications
- Especially antihypertensives, statins, antiplatelets, diabetes mellitus medications
- Allergies

Family history
- First degree relative with cardiovascular disease

Social history
- Smoking history
- Diet and exercise

 NB In reality, ulcers never fall neatly into one category – mixed ulcers are common, e.g. a neuropathic ulcer may be painful if it has a large enough arterial (ischaemic) component.

OSCE Key Learning Points

✔ Establishing the patient's background will often inform you as to the cause of the ulcer before examining it – e.g. if a patient has known chronic varicose vein disease, and no cardiovascular disease risk factors, the ulcer is likely due to venous insufficiency (without even asking any questions about the ulcer itself)

33 Loin pain

> **Definition:** Pain in either flank.

Differentials

- *Common*: renal calculi, pyelonephritis, infected obstructed kidney, urinary tract infection (UTI), muskuloskeletal
- *Rare*: renal tumour, papillary necrosis, glomerulonephritis, retroperitoneal fibrosis (e.g. caused by medications such as methyldopa and bromocriptine), dissecting aortic aneurysm, loin pain haematuria syndrome

History

 NB Infection control measures.

History of presenting complaint
- Onset of pain (sudden or chronic)
- Character of pain (sharp, dull, colicky)
- Constant or intermittent
- Radiation of pain (loin to groin)
- Exacerbating features (e.g. movement)
- Relieving factors (e.g. analgesia or rest)
- Associated symptoms:
  - Nausea and vomiting
  - Fever/rigours
  - Haematuria – if present, is it painful (e.g. renal calculi) or painless (renal tumour)
  - Dysuria

Medical Student Survival Skills: History Taking and Communication Skills, First Edition.
Philip Jevon and Steve Odogwu.
© 2020 John Wiley & Sons Ltd. Published 2020 by John Wiley & Sons Ltd.
Companion website: www.wiley.com/go/jevon/medicalstudent

- Urinary frequency
- History of back pain
- Weight loss

Past medical and surgical history
- Previous UTIs or kidney infections
- Diabetes mellitus, hypertension, hypercholesterolaemia, or any other illnesses
- Any previous surgery – especially urological, gynaecological, or abdominal

Medications and allergies
- Current medications
- Analgesia overuse
- Methyldopa
- Bromocriptine
- Recent antibiotics
- Allergies

Family history
- Family history of renal calculi (risk is doubled with a positive family history)

Social history
- Who patient lives with at home
- Smoking and alcohol
- Diet
- Occupation

OSCE Key Learning Points

✔ In particular, remember to ask about loin to groin pain and fever

 NB With any history of fever and loin pain, an obstructed infected kidney needs to be ruled out as it has the potential to be life-threatening.

 Common misinterpretations and pitfalls

Establish exact site of pain and use direct questions to help rule in/out specific diagnoses.

34 Loss of memory

Definition: Loss of memory (also called amnesia) is where the patient loses the ability to remember information and events they would normally be able to recall.

Differentials

- *Common*: depression, stress, head injury, stroke, age-related impairment, medications, e.g. sedatives and parkinsonian drugs, alcohol use, sleep impairment, dementia, e.g. Alzheimer's, delirium (Table 34.1)
- *Rare*: endocrine disorders, e.g. hypothyroidism, tumours, human immuno-deficiency virus (HIV)

History

 NB Infection control measures, introduction, and consent.

History of presenting complaint
- Establish type of symptom:
  - Amnesia (deficit in memory, e.g. everyday events)
  - Agnosia (unable to recognise objects/people)
  - Aphasia (loss of ability to understand speech/express), e.g. do people understand what you are saying?
  - Apraxia (loss of ability to perform complex coordinated movements), e.g. do you have problems dressing?
  - Mood or personality changes
  - Hallucinations and delusions

Medical Student Survival Skills: History Taking and Communication Skills, First Edition.
Philip Jevon and Steve Odogwu.
© 2020 John Wiley & Sons Ltd. Published 2020 by John Wiley & Sons Ltd.
Companion website: www.wiley.com/go/jevon/medicalstudent

Table 34.1 Differences between dementia and delirium.

Dementia	Delirium
Global cognitive disorder	Global cognitive disorder
Gradual onset	Acute onset
Lasts months to years	Lasts days to weeks
Normal consciousness	Fluctuations in consciousness
Impaired memory	Impaired memory
Insomnia in some cases	Reversal of sleep–wake cycle

- Sleep disturbances, e.g. reversal of sleep–wake cycle.
- Inappropriate behaviour, e.g. sexual disinhibition
- Duration of symptoms
- Any triggers/stressors
- Gradual progression or stepwise, e.g. slow and steady or deteriorates then stabilises
- Effect on activities of daily living, e.g. cooking, washing, shopping
- Screen for depression
- Head injury

 NB Get a collateral history.

Past medical history
- Vascular risk factors, e.g. cholesterol, blood pressure, smoker, previous stroke

Family history
- Dementia – especially if <65 years
- Past psychiatric history
- Depression
- Other mental health illness

Medications and allergies
- Current medications, e.g. sedatives and hypnotics
- Allergies

Social history
- Support available
- Who patient lives with – any social issues

- Smoking and alcohol
- Assess carers' needs – relationship to patient, amount of care needed, stress
- Find out what help is needed, expectation of service, awareness of voluntary organisations, and understanding of patient's illness

Risk assessment
- Assess risk to self and others, e.g. wandering and aggression
- Perform the Mini Mental State Examination (MMSE)

OSCE Key Learning Points

✔ Ensure the social history and risk are assessed

 NB Collateral history.

35 Low mood

> **Definition:** A persistent feeling of hopelessness or worthlessness.

Differentials

- *Common*: depression, stress-related disorders (bereavement/adjustment disorders), secondary to psychical illness
- *Rare*: medication or illicit substance side effects, other psychiatric illness (bipolar disorder), endocrine (hypothyroidism/menopause)

History

 NB Ensure your own personal safety (i.e. sit nearer the door).

History of presenting complaint
- Ask about the course of the low mood (onset, diurnal variation, triggers)
- Explore what happened prior to low mood onset (precipitating factors)
- Psychological symptoms: anhedonia (diminished pleasure in activities), hopelessness, guilt, worthlessness, anxiety
- Biological: sleep, appetite, weight loss, fatigue, psychomotor agitation/retardation, poor concentration, poor libido
- Social: coping strategies, children (safeguarding), occupation (sick leave), hobbies, other responsibilities
- Explore for delusions (paranoia, poverty, grandiose), hallucinations (auditory, olfactory, visual), thought disorder (insertion/withdrawal)
- Ask about pre-morbid personality
- Enquire about other physical symptoms (e.g. of anaemia, endocrine disease)

Medical Student Survival Skills: History Taking and Communication Skills, First Edition.
Philip Jevon and Steve Odogwu.
© 2020 John Wiley & Sons Ltd. Published 2020 by John Wiley & Sons Ltd.
Companion website: www.wiley.com/go/jevon/medicalstudent

- Ask about current thoughts or plans of self-harm/suicide
- Ask about thought or plans to harm others and any relevant forensic history

Past medical history
- Any concurrent illnesses (acute or chronic)
- Past psychiatric history (especially duration of previous depressive periods and any manic episodes)
- Previous self-harm/suicide attempts
- If time, could explore personal history and childhood

Medications and allergies
- Current medications, antidepressants
- Allergies

Family history
- Any family members with similar symptoms
- Any psychiatric illnesses in relatives

Social history
- Who patient lives with (supportive partner/domestic abuse/are they a carer?)
- Smoking, alcohol, and drug misuse

OSCE Key Learning Points

✔ In particular, remember to ask about thoughts, and history, of self-harm, suicide, and harm to others

 NB Often 'low mood' presents with anxiety (see Chapter 6).

 Uncommon presentations

Depression may present with only biological symptoms.

 Common misinterpretations and pitfalls

Not all 'low mood' is depression, remember to think about other psychiatric illness (bipolar disorder) and physical illnesses.

36 Lumps and bumps

Differentials

These depend on the anatomical location.

Head, neck, and extremities
- *Common*: inflammation (parotid, lymph nodes), lipoma, cysts (sebaceous, thyroid), skin cancers (basal or squamous cell carcinoma, melanoma)
- *Rare*: tumour (thyroid, parotid, acoustic neuroma), cervical rib, subclavian/popliteal aneurysm

Thorax, abdomen, and pelvis
- *Common*: hernia (inguinal>femoral), lipoma, seborrhoeic keratosis, epididymitis, breast cysts/fibroadenoma, abscesses
- *Rare*: tumours (breast, testicle), genital (varicocele, Bartholin's cyst, hydrocele), aortic aneurysm

History

History of presenting complaint
- Onset – when did you notice it or /what made you notice it?
- Events – trauma/bites/recent illnesses
- Pain – use SOCRATES (see Chapter 8)
- Changes – in colour, shape, size, temperature, pulsatile
- More – lumps elsewhere?
- Healing – has it ever disappeared or is it reducible
- Function – any limitations (swallowing/hearing/salivating); bowel/urine habit
- Discharge – bleeding/pus/slough

Medical Student Survival Skills: History Taking and Communication Skills, First Edition.
Philip Jevon and Steve Odogwu.
© 2020 John Wiley & Sons Ltd. Published 2020 by John Wiley & Sons Ltd.
Companion website: www.wiley.com/go/jevon/medicalstudent

Past medical and surgical history
- Diabetes
- Obesity
- Chronic obstructive pulmonary disease, chronic cough
- Thyroid disease
- Connective tissue disease
- Any previous surgery – especially hernia repairs and incision and drainage
- Any biopsies

Medications and allergies
- Current medications – especially thyroid and diabetic
- History of antibiotics
- Allergies

Family history
- Cancers – try not to alarm patient
- Congenital malformations

Social history
- Occupation – any sports or heavy lifting involved
- General hygiene
- Smoking and alcohol
- Sun exposure – tanning beds, sun cream use, etc.

OSCE Key Learning Points

✔ Do not forget functionality and effect on lifestyle; sun exposure in suspected skin cancers (mention prevention advice in management); previous lumps and surgeries (incisional hernias); and that groin and axilla abscesses can form after shaving (trauma)

 Common misinterpretations and pitfalls

Bleeding and changes in skin lesions are highly suspicious of cancer; skin cancer can affect any part of the body and are increasing in prevalence.

(37) Melaena

> **Definition:** Passing dark motions caused by bleeding from the upper gastrointestinal (GI) tract; blood appearance is altered by digestive enzymes.

Differentials

Upper GI bleeds are usually in the oesophagus, stomach, or duodenum.
- *Common*: bleeding peptic/duodenal ulcer, upper GI malignancy, bleeding oesophageal varices, Mallory–Weiss tears

 NB May be mistaken for the black stools of iron supplementation.

History

History of presenting complaint
- Description of the stool
  - Black
  - Sticky
  - 'Tar-like'
  - Offensive
- Number of episodes
- Any associated symptoms
  - Epigastric pain – SOCRATES approach (see Chapter 8) (radiation, exacerbated by certain foods, worse at night, etc.)
  - Reflux/heartburn
- Any vomiting

Medical Student Survival Skills: History Taking and Communication Skills, First Edition.
Philip Jevon and Steve Odogwu.
© 2020 John Wiley & Sons Ltd. Published 2020 by John Wiley & Sons Ltd.
Companion website: www.wiley.com/go/jevon/medicalstudent

- Is there haematemesis
  - 'Coffee-ground'
  - Fresh blood in vomit
  - Clots seen
- Red flag symptoms
- Weight loss
- Night sweats
- Progressive dysphagia
- Anorexia
- Any suggestion of circulatory compromise or massive haemorrhage
- Light-headedness/dizziness
- Postural hypotension
- Chest pain/angina
- Dyspnoea
- Palpitations
- Collapse
- Lethargy

Past medical history
- Gastro-oesophageal reflux disease
- Peptic ulcer disease
- Alcohol excess – may cause varices
- Arthritis
- Musculoskeletal pain
- Chronic pain
- Asthma/chronic obstructive pulmonary disease
- Skin conditions (e.g. eczema)

NB Consider any hints suggesting recent non-steroidal anti-inflammatory drug (NSAID) or steroid use – patient may have recently completed a course, and will not consider this in current medications.

Family history
- GI cancers

Medications
- Steroids
- NSAIDs
- Aspirin
- Iron supplements
- Proton pump inhibitors (PPIs)
- Antacids

Social history
- Smoking
- Alcohol consumption (past and present)

OSCE Key Learning Points

✔ Confirm risk factors for upper GI bleed
✔ Do not forget red flag symptoms for malignancy – weight loss, fever/night sweats, dysphagia, and anorexia

38 Menorrhagia

> **Definition:** Heavy regular menstrual bleeding that is affecting the biological, social, or psychological aspects of a woman's life. It is also defined as $>80\,ml$ blood loss per menstrual cycle.

Differentials

- *Common*: dysfunctional uterine bleeding (DUB), endometrial polyps or fibroids, infection, iatrogenic (hormonal contraceptives or replacement)
- *Rare*: bleeding from undiagnosed pregnancy, clotting disorders, endometrial cancer, endometriosis (more likely to cause cyclical pain)

History

 NB Always consider *pregnancy* when taking a gynaecological history.

History of presenting complaint
- Determine volume of menses; number of changes of sanitary product per day, flooding, clotting
- Associated pelvic/abdominal pain and relation to menses
- Regularity and duration of menstrual cycle and menses
- Last menstrual period (LMP)
- When did it start (since first period/since pregnancy, etc.)
- Any intermenstrual, post-coital, or post-menopausal bleeding
- Vaginal discharge
- Dyspareunia

Medical Student Survival Skills: History Taking and Communication Skills, First Edition.
Philip Jevon and Steve Odogwu.
© 2020 John Wiley & Sons Ltd. Published 2020 by John Wiley & Sons Ltd.
Companion website: www.wiley.com/go/jevon/medicalstudent

- Other bruising/bleeding
- Weight loss/fever
- Abdominal bloating
- Symptoms of anaemia
- Possibility of pregnancy (contraception, sexual partners)

Past medical and surgical history
- Age of menarche
- Previous gynaecological problems
- Cervical sampling results
- Use of hormonal contraceptives and hormone replacement therapy (HRT)
- Gynaecological cancers and cancer treatment
- Known clotting disorders
- Any previous surgery – especially gynaecological or abdominal

Medications and allergies
- Current medications
- Warfarin use
- Contraception (including non-oral formulations)
- Allergies

Family history
- Gynaecological problems including cancer

Social history
- Determine the impact of the bleeding on the patient's life
- Smoking, alcohol, and illicit substance use

OSCE Key Learning Points

✔ In particular, remember to ask about the social impact of the bleeding

 Uncommon presentations

Anaemia, as a result of menorrhagia, may be the presenting complaint.

NB Any intermenstrual, post-coital, and post-menopausal bleeding should be fully investigated.

 Common misinterpretations and pitfalls

Women have different views on how much bleeding to expect, try to clarify their loss in terms of sanitary wear usage (e.g. pads per hour/day).

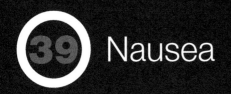

39 Nausea

Definition: A feeling of wanting to vomit.

Differentials

- *Common*: gastroenteritis (viral and bacterial), food poisoning, motion sickness, pregnancy, surgical (e.g. peptic ulcer disease)
- *Rare*: iatrogenic (e.g. cytotoxic drugs, antibiotics), migraine, middle ear disorders, myocardial infarction

History

 NB Infection control measures if associated with diarrhoea.

History of presenting complaint
- Nature: retching, heaving
- When it started
- Timing: constant, intermittent
- Is patient aware of any potential triggers, e.g. car travel
- Associated dyspepsia, vomiting, diarrhoea, pain (further history on these symptoms will be required)
- Recent dietary history
- Fever
- Relieving factors
- Other associated symptoms: central nervous system – headache, dizziness, tremor; urinary – dysuria, frequency
- Recent foreign travel
- Close contacts with similar symptoms

Medical Student Survival Skills: History Taking and Communication Skills, First Edition.
Philip Jevon and Steve Odogwu.
© 2020 John Wiley & Sons Ltd. Published 2020 by John Wiley & Sons Ltd.
Companion website: www.wiley.com/go/jevon/medicalstudent

Past medical history
- History of reflux disease
- Migraine
- Malignancy (especially if undergoing chemotherapy currently)
- Females – pregnancy
- Ischaemic heart disease

Medications and allergies
- Current medications (any anti-emetics tried?)
- Recent antibiotics
- Allergies

Social history
- Occupation
- Relationship status
- Any dependents, e.g. children or elderly family
- Smoking and alcohol (withdrawal)
- Recent foreign travel

OSCE Key Learning Points

✔ Nausea often has clear identifiable triggers
✔ Most commonly associated with other symptoms, e.g. vomiting and abdominal pain. Identify them early to allow yourself time to enquire about them further

 NB Nausea in isolation is a common symptom associated with stress, fatigue, etc., it is a 'functional' symptom, often with no medical cause.

 Common misinterpretations and pitfalls

Pregnancy is a very common cause of nausea – a must-ask question in females of reproductive age!

40 Numbness and weakness

> **Definition:**
> - *Weakness* is clinical symptom suggestive of a motor deficit.
> - *Numbness* is clinical symptom suggestive of a sensory deficit.

Differentials

- *Central* (upper motor neuron): cerebral vascular accident (CVA), cord compression, cauda equina, multiple sclerosis (MS), trauma, central nervous system neoplasia, haematoma, spinal abscess
- *Peripheral* (lower motor neuron): diabetes mellitus (DM), vitamin B_{12}/folate deficiency, alcohol excess, renal failure, hypothyroidism, motor neuron disease, nerve entrapment, inflammatory (Gullian–Barré, systemic lupus erythematosus)

History

 NB Think about medical emergencies (cord compression) and indication for thrombolysis (CVA).

History of presenting complaint
- Onset – get exact time
- Sudden or gradual
- Progression of symptoms – worsening, static, or improving
- Other neurological symptoms such as visual disturbance, headache, and dysphasia.
- Loss/reduced bladder or bowel control
- Associated pain, neck stiffness, rashes, recent behavioural change

Medical Student Survival Skills: History Taking and Communication Skills, First Edition.
Philip Jevon and Steve Odogwu.
© 2020 John Wiley & Sons Ltd. Published 2020 by John Wiley & Sons Ltd.
Companion website: www.wiley.com/go/jevon/medicalstudent

- Recent illness, trauma, bleeding, thrombolysis
- Any weight loss, fever, or night sweats

Past medical and surgical history
- Previous neurology – intracranial pathology, migraines, epilepsy, MS, psychiatric disorder
- Cardiovascular history – transient ischaemic attack (TIA)/strokes, DM, ischaemic heart disease, hypertension, atrial fibrillation
- Bleeding disorder – clotting problems, haemophilia, liver failure, gastrointestinal bleeds
- Any history of malignancy
- Invasive procedures/surgery – thrombolysis

Medications and allergies
- Current medications
- Anticoagulation
- Antipsychotics
- Allergies

Social history
- Independence and disability living allowance (DLA)
- Alcohol intake
- Smoking
- Recent foreign travel
- Dietary intake

Family history
- MI and stoke/TIA
- Nerve or muscle problems

OSCE Key Learning Points

✔ In particular, establish the exact start of symptoms and progression, and suggest the need to perform both neurological and cardiovascular system examinations

NB Consider thrombolysis in ischaemic stroke < 4.5 hours from start of symptoms. It is vital to rule out early on any medical emergencies such as cord compression and cauda equina.

 Common misinterpretations and pitfalls

Determine whether weakness or numbness is localised, indicating focal neurology, or generalised, suggesting more systemic pathology.

41 Paediatrics: Diarrhoea

Definition: Loose or liquid stool at increased frequency compared with normal.

Differentials

- *Common*: gastroenteritis (viral, bacterial, parasitic), dietary protein intolerances, post gastroenteritis, lactose intolerance, irritable bowel syndrome, toddler diarrhoea, coeliac disease, inflammatory bowel disease (IBD), antibiotic use
- *Rare*: malabsorption secondary to liver, bowel, or pancreatic disorders, primary lactose intolerance

History

NB Remember to direct questions to the child if old enough and involve the child fully in the consultation. Establish carer's identity and document that they were present when taking the history. It is important to document the child's age and weight.

History of presenting complaint
- Duration of symptoms
- Consistency of stool and what stool is like – offensive and difficult to flush, containing undigested vegetables
- Number of episodes per day
- Any blood, pus, or mucous in stool or any PR bleeding
- Is the blood jelly like or fresh red

Medical Student Survival Skills: History Taking and Communication Skills, First Edition.
Philip Jevon and Steve Odogwu.
© 2020 John Wiley & Sons Ltd. Published 2020 by John Wiley & Sons Ltd.
Companion website: www.wiley.com/go/jevon/medicalstudent

- Oral intake – fluids and food in the last 24 hours
- What is the child's diet normally like
- Any vomiting
- Urine output – how many wet nappies in 24 hours/times per day going to toilet
- Any abdominal pain – SOCRATES approach (see Chapter 8)
- Any history of diarrhoea before this episode or altered bowel habit
- Systemic symptoms including fevers or rashes
- Any abnormal or different food recently
- Is the child putting on weight and growing well
- Any irritability or abdominal distension
- Any joint pains
- Any oral ulcers

Past medical and surgical history
- Obstetric history:
  - Mode of delivery
  - Gestation at birth
  - Birth weight
  - Any problems during pregnancy
  - Any problems soon after birth – was the patient admitted to the neonatal unit, and if so details
- Any previous hospital admissions or medical conditions – including liver disease or exocrine pancreatic disorder, e.g. cystic fibrosis, episodes of uveitis, arthritis, spondylitis
- Any operations – particularly bowel resection

Medications and allergies
- Any regular medications or access to others' medications at home
- Recent use of antibiotics
- Any allergies
- Are immunisations up to date

Family history
- Ethnic origin
- Family tree
- Consanguinity
- Family history of bowel disturbances, IBD, or coeliac disease
- Any one at home unwell with diarrhoea

Social history

- Who lives at home and family make up, hobbies/interests, is the child happy at home
- Is the child at school or nursery – anyone there unwell with diarrhoea, is the child happy at school
- Any recent travel abroad, any contaminated drinking water or unsanitary preparation of food, exposure to freshwater streams and pools
- Development – key developmental milestones, any concerns

OSCE Key Learning Points

✔ It is important to gauge the input and output of the child to assess dehydration, as well as to clinically examine for dehydration status

✔ Ask about travel, infectious contacts, and different or abnormal food

 NB It is fairly common for an infant to have loose stool so ask what stool is like compared with normal.

 Common misinterpretations and pitfalls

Always ask about what the child's stool is normally like and how it has changed – different people have different perceptions of diarrhoea. If talking to child do not use medical terminology and explain in simple terms so they understand.

42 Paediatrics: Convulsions/seizures

Definition: Sudden disturbance of neurological function caused by an abnormal neuronal discharge, often manifesting in involuntary muscular movements, sensory disturbances, and altered consciousness.

Differentials

- *Common*: febrile convulsion, breath-holding attack, reflex anoxic seizure, syncope, meningitis/encephalitis, epilepsy, head trauma, metabolic disturbances (including hypoglycaemia, hypocalcemia, hypo/hypernatraemia)
- *Rare*: cardiac arrhythmia, pseudoseizures/fabricated illness, neurodegenerative disorders, neurocutaneous syndromes, cerebral tumour, poisoning

History

 NB Remember to direct questions to the child if old enough and involve the child fully in the consultation. Establish carer's identity and document that they were present when taking history. It is important to document the child's age and weight.

History of presenting complaint
- Ask parent/carer to explain what happened – what did they witness, any video
- What were they doing immediately before the seizure
- Was the child hot immediately prior to the seizure, was the temperature measured
- Determine if seizure was focal or generalised (affecting one part of body or whole body)

Medical Student Survival Skills: History Taking and Communication Skills, First Edition.
Philip Jevon and Steve Odogwu.
© 2020 John Wiley & Sons Ltd. Published 2020 by John Wiley & Sons Ltd.
Companion website: www.wiley.com/go/jevon/medicalstudent

- Did it start focal and then secondarily generalise
- Determine if seizure was simple or complex (any altered consciousness)
- Any tongue biting, incontinence, eye rolling
- Was any intervention required to terminate the seizure, e.g. midazolam
- Determine if there was a post-ictal phase (time afterwards when child was not their normal self)
- Determine roughly how long the episode lasted – seizure and post ictal-phase
- Are they back to normal now? What's different?
- Determine if there was any colour change in the child and what happened just before seizure – any triggers (flashing lights, breath holding, cold, fright, etc.)
- Any previous episodes
- Any preceding illness – fever, coryza, sore throat, pulling at ears, reduced oral intake, lethargy, irritability, change in behaviour, etc.
- Any history of trauma to head – before or during seizure
- Reported headaches, vomiting, lethargy
- Other neurological symptoms including reduced strength, altered sensation, disturbed vision, atypical behaviour, impaired balance or gait

Past medical and surgical history
- Obstetric history:
  - Mode of delivery
  - Gestation at birth
  - Birth weight
  - Any problems during pregnancy
  - Any problems soon after birth – was the patient admitted to the neonatal unit, and if so details – any history of cerebral damage perinatally, e.g. congenital infection, hypoxic-ischaemic encephalopathy, intraventricular haemorrhage/ischaemia
- Any previous hospital admissions or medical conditions including epilepsy, any history of cerebral malformation, or cerebral vascular events
- Any operations

Medications and allergies
- Any regular medications – has the child ever been on antiepileptic medication, do they have access to other medications
- Any allergies
- Are immunisations up to date

Family history
- Family tree
- Consanguinity
- Family history of epilepsy or febrile convulsions
- Any one at home unwell

Social history
- Who lives at home and family make up, hobbies/interests, is the child happy at home
- Is the child at school or nursery, is the child happy at school
- Development – key developmental milestones, any regression, any concerns

OSCE Key Learning Points

✔ Ask the witness open questions about seizure – it is important to get an accurate history as this forms a big part of the diagnosis

 NB If a child has had a febrile convulsion, it is important to think about the source of the infection.

 Common misinterpretations and pitfalls

Seizures do not always equal epilepsy and diagnosis of epilepsy cannot be made after one seizure. Ask parents about previous episodes and whether been on antiepileptic medication to check whether has diagnosis of epilepsy.

43 Paediatrics: Difficulty in breathing

Definition: Problems with breathing including rapid respiratory rate, poor oxygenation, and noisy breathing.

Differentials

- *Common*: asthma, croup, bronchiolitis, pneumonia, pertussis, upper respiratory track infection (URTI), congenital heart disease
- *Rare*: epiglottitis, bacterial tracheitis, laryngomalacia, anaphylaxis, foreign body inhalation, congenital respiratory anomalies such as vascular ring and laryngeal web, hypocalcaemia, tumour

History

 NB Remember to direct questions to the child if old enough and involve the child fully in the consultation. Establish carer's identity and document that they were present when taking history. It is important to document the child's age and weight.

History of presenting complaint
- Speed and time of onset – sudden or gradual, day or night time
- Noisy breathing – inspiratory, expiratory, or both
- Wheeze (see Chapter 46)
- Stridor present – harsh or soft, on crying or at rest; hoarseness
- Cough – nature of cough – barking, sharp and dry, paroxysmal/spasmodic
- Respiratory distress – indrawing of chest, head bobbing, tracheal tug, nasal flaring, abdominal breathing

Medical Student Survival Skills: History Taking and Communication Skills, First Edition.
Philip Jevon and Steve Odogwu.
© 2020 John Wiley & Sons Ltd. Published 2020 by John Wiley & Sons Ltd.
Companion website: www.wiley.com/go/jevon/medicalstudent

- Is the child able to speak and/or swallow, any drooling
- Is the child able to tolerate food and drink, any difficulty in breathing or sweating when feeding
- Any breathlessness on exertion
- Is the child gaining weight well
- Any fevers – low or high grade and duration
- Any coryzal symptoms, sore throat, pulling at ears
- Any lethargy/feeling generally unwell
- Any chest, abdominal, or neck pain?
- Any episodes of apnoea (where the child stops breathing) – any colour change, length and number of episodes
- Any history of playing with foreign body or seeing foreign body in mouth
- Any previous episodes of difficulty in breathing
- Any recurrent respiratory infections
- Any previous stridor from birth

Past medical and surgical history
- Obstetric history
  - Mode of delivery
  - Gestation at birth
  - Birth weight
  - Any problems during pregnancy
  - Any problems soon after birth – was the patient admitted to the neonatal unit, and if so details
  - Did the patient have chronic lung disease – often go home on oxygen
  - Did the patient have any congenital cardiac abnormality
- Any previous hospital admissions or medical conditions
- Any operations

Medications and allergies
- Any regular medications
- Any allergies
- Are immunisations up to date

Family history
- Family tree
- Consanguinity
- Family history of babies born with heart murmurs or problems
- Anyone else at home unwell

Social history
- Who lives at home and family make up, hobbies/interests, is the child happy at home
- Is the child at school or nursery, is the child happy at school
- Anyone at home smoking
- Pets
- Development – key developmental milestones, any concerns

OSCE Key Learning Points

✔ Chest, abdominal, or neck pain can be a sign of pleural irritation and can be present in pneumonia

✔ Children who are premature with chronic lung disease or have congenital cardiac abnormality are more at risk of bronchiolitis with increased severity

 NB Do not attempt to examine or upset children with high temperature, stridor, or possible airway compromise.

44 Paediatrics: Non-specific unwell neonate

You will often be asked to see a neonate who is just 'not right' – this encompasses a wide range of symptoms including abnormal behaviour and problems with feeding. There is a long list of differentials.

Differentials

- *Common*: sepsis, meningitis, dehydration, jaundice, hypoglycaemia, necrotising enterocolitis, volvulus, intussusception, pyloric stenosis
- *Rare*: inborn errors of metabolism, congenital heart disease (e.g. duct-dependent disease), myocarditis, pericarditis or cardiomyopathy, cardiac dysrhythmia such as supraventricular tachycardia, non-accidental injury, congenital adrenal hyperplasia, severe anaemia, hypothyroidism, neoplasm

History

NB Be vigilant for non-accidental injury. Look for suspicious elements such as delays in presentation, inconsistent history between care givers and repeated histories, inappropriate carer's response (e.g. unconcerned/aggressive), and signs not in keeping with the clinical history or developmental stage of the infant.

History of presenting complaint
- Ask parent/midwife to explain what is not right about infant
- How is the infant feeding – what type, how much it normally takes and how often, what is the feeding like currently, is the infant waking spontaneously for feeds
- Any sweating during feeding

Medical Student Survival Skills: History Taking and Communication Skills, First Edition.
Philip Jevon and Steve Odogwu.
© 2020 John Wiley & Sons Ltd. Published 2020 by John Wiley & Sons Ltd.
Companion website: www.wiley.com/go/jevon/medicalstudent

- Has there been any vomiting
- Any abdominal distension, any signs of discomfort or pain
- Has the baby been opening its bowels as normal, any diarrhoea or blood, mucous or tissue in stool
- How many wet nappies has the baby had in the last 24 hours (sign of urine output)
- Is the baby maintaining its own temperature or feels warm
- Has the baby seemed lethargic or irritable
- Has the baby been jittery or unsettled
- Has the baby had any symptoms/signs of respiratory distress, any apneoas
- Has the baby been jaundiced, colour of urine and stool
- Has the baby had any rash or mottling of skin or bruises or rashes that do not disappear on pressure, any blueness particularly around lips
- Has the baby had any hypotonia or seizures
- Is the baby gaining weight appropriately
- Any swelling of limbs or joints

Past medical and surgical history
- Obstetric history
  - Mode of delivery and gestation at birth
  - Did the infant receive prophylactic vitamin K
  - Birth weight and centile – did the baby have intrauterine growth retardation or macrosomy
  - Any problems during pregnancy
- Ask specifically about risks for infection such as pre-labour or prolonged rupture of membranes, maternal group B streptococcal (GBS) infection or previous baby with GBS infection, recent infection in mother causing pyrexia, or signs of chorioamnionitis
- Ask specifically if there was any maternal diabetes during pregnancy and how well it was controlled
- Does the mother have any medical conditions (including endocrine problems or systemic diseases, e.g. systemic lupus erythematosus) and was she on any medications during the pregnancy
- Were antenatal scans normal, were any extra scans needed
- Any problems soon after birth – was the condition good at birth, did the baby require any resuscitation, was there meconium present at birth
- Was the patient admitted to the neonatal unit and if so details why, what was done, length of stay including whether they had any surgery
- Any abnormalities/signs of dysmorphism on baby check

- Any readmissions after birth if coming in from community
- Was the Guthrie test performed

Medications and allergies
- Has the baby had any medications
- Any known allergies

Family history
- Family tree
- Consanguinity
- Family history of unwell babies including still births or early neonatal deaths or babies with heart murmurs
- Any one at home unwell at present

Social history
- Who lives at home and family make up

OSCE Key Learning Points

✔ It is important in neonates to get a good maternal history, antenatal history, delivery history, and immediate postnatal history to inform diagnosis
✔ Sweating when feeding can be a sign of congenital heart disease

 Common misinterpretations and pitfalls

Do not ignore a parent or midwife if they say a neonate is 'not right' as neonates can present with non-specific symptoms for serious diseases. Have a high index of suspicion for sepsis, which may be insidious.

45 Paediatrics: Vomiting

Definition: Forceful ejection of gastric contents.

Differentials

- *Common*: Gastro-oesophageal reflux, overfeeding, gastroenteritis, infection (including URTI, UTI, meningitis, and pertussis), dietary protein intolerances
- *Less common*: pyloric stenosis, appendicitis, intestinal obstruction (including malrotation, volvulus, intussusception, atresia, strangulated hernia), diabetic ketoacidosis, migraine
- *Rare*: raised intracranial pressure, peptic ulceration, *Helicobacter pylori* infection, pregnancy, torsion of testis, inborn errors of metabolism, renal failure, congenital adrenal hyperplasia, hepatitis A

History

 NB Remember to direct questions to the child if old enough and involve the child fully in the consultation. Establish carer's identity and document that they were present when taking the history. It is important to document the child's age and weight.

History of presenting complaint
- Duration of symptoms
- Vomiting or posseting (non-forceful return of milk in small amounts, which often accompanies wind) or regurgitation (non-forceful return of milk in larger amounts, which is more frequent), relationship of vomiting to meals
- Typical dietary intake

Medical Student Survival Skills: History Taking and Communication Skills, First Edition.
Philip Jevon and Steve Odogwu.
© 2020 John Wiley & Sons Ltd. Published 2020 by John Wiley & Sons Ltd.
Companion website: www.wiley.com/go/jevon/medicalstudent

129

- Number of episodes, do they follow a pattern (e.g. the same time each month)
- Is it projectile
- Colour of vomit – is it bilious (green), faeculent, or blood stained
- Is the vomiting after coughing bouts
- Able to keep down fluids and/or food and what has oral intake been like
- If infant, what milk do they have, how much do they normally have, and how often and how much are they having now
- How many wet nappies were there in last 24 hours or how many times has the child gone to the toilet
- Have bowels been open as normal, is there any diarrhoea
- Is the child excessively thirsty or hungry
- Any signs of abdominal pain (including drawing legs up into belly) – SOCRATES approach (see Chapter 8)
- Is the child gaining weight properly, any weight loss, child's current weight and centile
- Fevers
- Any dysuria, polyuria, or unilateral abdominal/flank pain
- Cough, coryza, sore throat, pulling at ears
- Any signs of raised intracranial pressure – chronic headache, fatigue, weakness, weight loss, and early-morning vomiting?

Past medical and surgical history
- Obstetric history
  - Mode of delivery
  - Gestation at birth
  - Birth weight
  - Any problems during pregnancy
  - Any problems soon after birth – was the patient admitted to the neonatal unit and if so details
- Any previous hospital admissions or medical conditions – including neuromuscular disorders and diabetes
- Any operations – particularly on oesophagus or diaphragm, e.g. oesophageal atresia or diaphragmatic hernia

Medications and allergies
- Any regular medications or access to others' medications
- Any allergies
- Are immunisations up to date

Family history
- Family tree including still births or deaths in infancy
- Consanguinity
- Family history of pyloric stenosis
- Any one at home unwell

Social history
- Who lives at home and family make up, hobbies/interests, is the child happy at home
- Is the child at school or nursery – anyone there unwell with vomiting, is the child happy at school
- Any recent travel abroad, any contaminated drinking water or unsanitary food preparation
- Development – key developmental milestones, any concerns

OSCE Key Learning Points

✔ Gastro-oesophageal reflux is common in the first year of life and infants have an increased risk if they have neuromuscular disorders or have had surgery on the oesophagus or diaphragm
✔ Pyloric stenosis presents between 2 and 7 weeks of age and is more common in first born boys with a maternal family history

---

 Common misinterpretations and pitfalls

Parents can often overestimate the amount of vomiting by the child. Ask the parent if the child vomits to show the nurse so that an accurate record of the amount and colour of the vomit can be made.

46 Paediatrics: Wheeze

Definition: Musical expiratory whistling sound when breathing which can be audible or found on auscultation of chest signifying lower airway narrowing.

Differentials

- *Common*: acute exacerbation of asthma, viral-induced wheeze, bronchiolitis, pneumonia
- *Rare*: cystic fibrosis, bronchiectasis, pulmonary oedema, anaphylaxis

History

NB Remember to direct questions to the child if old enough and involve the child fully in the consultation. Establish carer's identity and document that they were present when taking the history. It is important to document the child's age and weight.

History of presenting complaint
- Is it wheeze – see Chapter 43 if is stridor or hoarseness
- Duration of symptoms and speed and time of onset
- Difficulty in breathing or signs of respiratory distress – indrawing of chest
- Cough – dry or productive
- Coryzal symptoms, sore throat, or pulling at ears
- Fevers
- Has the child been generally unwell/lethargic
- Facial swelling, tongue swelling, or rash

Medical Student Survival Skills: History Taking and Communication Skills, First Edition.
Philip Jevon and Steve Odogwu.
© 2020 John Wiley & Sons Ltd. Published 2020 by John Wiley & Sons Ltd.
Companion website: www.wiley.com/go/jevon/medicalstudent

- Is the child able to talk and eat and drink as normal
- What has the child's oral intake been like
- Is the child growing and putting on weight normally
- If have an inhaler – was this given at home and did they have any relief from it
- Has the child had any previous episodes – any triggers (including viral infections or environmental stimuli such as pets and cigarette smoke), did they require hospital admission, what treatment did they have, have they ever been in an intensive care unit
- Any interval symptoms (symptoms between episodes) – any shortness of breath or wheeze during exercise, any nocturnal cough, perennial versus seasonal
- If asthmatic – what is the child's normal peak flow

Past medical and surgical history
- Obstetric history
  - Mode of delivery
  - Gestation at birth
  - Birth weight
  - Any problems during pregnancy
  - Any problems soon after birth – was the patient admitted to the neonatal unit and if so details such as ventilation
  - Did the patient have chronic lung disease – often go home on oxygen
  - Did the patient have any congenital cardiac abnormality
- Any previous hospital admissions or medical conditions – including atopy
- Any operations

Medications and allergies
- Any regular medications – ask specifically about adrenaline autoinjectors and inhalers. How often does the child use the salbutamol inhaler on average? Is their technique adequate? How concordant are they with treatment?
- Any allergies – suspected or confirmed
- Are immunisations up to date

Family history
- Family tree
- Consanguinity?
- Family history of atopy – asthma, eczema, hay fever
- Any one at home unwell – chronic condition or history of problematic chest disease

Social history
- Who lives at home and family make up, hobbies/interests, is the child happy at home
- Is the house owned or rented, any mould, any building work
- Is the child at school or nursery, is the child happy at school, number of days off school
- Are there emotional triggers to the symptoms
- Anyone at home smoking, if so, would they consider quitting
- Pets – do their symptoms improve when spending nights away from them
- Development – key developmental milestones, any concerns

OSCE Key Learning Points

✔ Wheeze does not always mean asthma – it is important to find out about previous episodes in order to see whether the child has asthma or not

✔ Ask about inhaler technique and concordance – most will not reliably take inhalers most of the time

 NB Young children are unable to expectorate sputum so will often have a dry cough.

 Common misinterpretations and pitfalls

Parents can have a different perception of wheeze to health professionals, so listen yourself if possible. Parents and professionals may label children as having asthma prematurely; explore how many previous episodes the child has had and what these are caused by, if they have any interval symptoms, and what inhalers they are on before reaching a conclusion as to their asthma status.

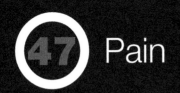

47 Pain

Definition: An unpleasant sensory and emotional experience which can be associated with actual or potential tissue damage, or described in terms of such damage.

History

History of presenting complaint
Use the SOCRATES approach:
- **S**ite
- **O**nset
- **C**haracter
- **R**adiation
- **A**ssociated symptoms and systems review as appropriate
- **T**iming
- **E**xacerbating/relieving factors
- **S**everity

Past medical and surgical history
- Any other medical problems
- Any recent acute illnesses
- Previous similar episodes and their investigation/management
- Any previous surgery – particularly around site of pain

Medications and allergies
- Current medications
- Allergies

Medical Student Survival Skills: History Taking and Communication Skills, First Edition.
Philip Jevon and Steve Odogwu.
© 2020 John Wiley & Sons Ltd. Published 2020 by John Wiley & Sons Ltd.
Companion website: www.wiley.com/go/jevon/medicalstudent

Family history
- Any illnesses that run in the family

Social history
- Who the patient lives with
- Are they able to continue normal activities, how much help do they require
- Occupation (consider occupational exposure to toxins or injury potential)
- Smoking, alcohol, illicit drug use (especially cocaine)
- Recent foreign travel

48 Palpitations

Definition: Conscious awareness of the heartbeat.

Differentials

- *Common*: physiological (stress, exercise), ectopic beats (atrial or ventricular), atrial fibrillation, drugs (caffeine, alcohol, salbutamol)
- *Rare*: thyrotoxicosis, anaemia, hypoglycaemia, other tachyarrhythmias (supraventricular/ventricular tachycardia)

History

NB Ask the patient to 'tap out' the rhythm – this can help you distinguish between a regular and irregular rhythm.

History of presenting complaint
- Site: neck or chest
- Onset: when they started (rest, exercise), sudden or gradual, previous episodes
- Timing: continuous/intermittent, frequency and duration (seconds/hours), time of day (night when quiet)
- Character: fast, slow, or isolated 'skipped beat'; rate – did patient check their own pulse; regular or irregular
- Tap out rhythm
- Missed beats
- Associated symptoms: chest pain, faintness, syncope/blackout/loss of consciousness, breathlessness

Medical Student Survival Skills: History Taking and Communication Skills, First Edition.
Philip Jevon and Steve Odogwu.
© 2020 John Wiley & Sons Ltd. Published 2020 by John Wiley & Sons Ltd.
Companion website: www.wiley.com/go/jevon/medicalstudent

- Tremor, recent weight loss
- Exacerbating/precipitating factors: any apparent triggers (alcohol, caffeine, exercise), does patient have history of anxiety (e.g. hyperventilation, panic attacks)
- Relieving/termination: spontaneous (sudden or gradual), manoeuvres (e.g. Valsalva)
- Severity

Past medical and surgical history
- Cardiac: ischaemic heart disease, hypertension, heart failure, valve disease
- Stroke
- Thyroid disease
- Previous heart surgery; does patient have a pacemaker
- Anxiety/depression
- Rheumatic fever as child
- Asthma

Medications and allergies
- Current medications – especially beta-blockers, digoxin
- Any anti-arrhythmics (e.g. amiodarone)
- Anticoagulants
- Caffeine intake
- Over the counter or herbal medications
- Allergies

Social history
- Occupation
- Physical fitness
- Smoking and alcohol
- Recreational drugs
- Interference with daily life

OSCE Key Learning Points

✔ A modified SOCRATES template can also be used when assessing palpitations

✔ Take time to assess the timing and character of the palpitations – this will help elicit if there is an underlying arrhythmia and also the type

NB Palpitations are common in all ages, but heart disease is more common in the elderly and anxiety or excessive caffeine use is more likely to be the cause in younger patients.

 Common misinterpretations and pitfalls

Do not miss red flag symptoms: chest pain, syncope, breathlessness – all point towards an underlying cardiac cause and will warrant further investigation.

(49) Paresthesia

Definition: Abnormal sensory symptoms typically characterised by tingling, prickling, pins and needles, or burning sensations. It can affect any part of the body innervated by sensory or afferent nerve fibres. Pathology affecting any part of the somatosensory pathway can cause a paresthesia.

Differentials

- *Central*: e.g. stroke, transient ischaemic attack, spinal cord compression
- *Peripheral*: e.g. diabetic neuropathy

History

NB The most common causes of paresthesias are peripheral neuropathies.

History of presenting complaint
- Thorough description of the sensation, e.g. burning, tingling
- Associated symptoms:
  - Loss in sensation
  - Pain – suggests inflammatory or ischaemic cause
  - Shooting pains – suggests nerve entrapment
- Onset:
  - Acute – vascular
  - Subacute – nerve entrapment

Medical Student Survival Skills: History Taking and Communication Skills, First Edition.
Philip Jevon and Steve Odogwu.
© 2020 John Wiley & Sons Ltd. Published 2020 by John Wiley & Sons Ltd.
Companion website: www.wiley.com/go/jevon/medicalstudent

- – Chronic – inherited neuropathy
- – Duration
- – Severity
- Location:
  - – Mononeuropathy
  - – Multiple mononeuropathy
  - – Polyneuropathy
  - – Plexopathy
- Precipitants, e.g. repetitive use or positioning in nerve entrapment
- Progression

Past medical and surgical history
- Diabetes
- Rheumatological conditions
- Previous cancers
- Previous infectious diseases
- Cardiovascular risk factors/strokes
- Previous trauma
- Any previous surgery – especially spinal or brain surgery

Medications and allergies
- Current and previous medications
- Allergies

Social history
- Alcohol history – previous or current abuse
- Diet – malnutrition or vegan diet
- Smoking – paraneoplastic syndromes
- Occupation – exposure to heavy metals, repetitive movement, or use of vibratory tools
- Sexual history – human immunodeficiency virus (HIV) neuropathy

Family history
- Inherited neuropathy

OSCE Key Learning Points

✔ Thorough evaluation of the pattern, precipitants, and associated symptoms of the paresthesia are the key to diagnosis

 Common misinterpretations and pitfalls

It is often difficult to describe vague symptom with a huge range of causes. Spending time on the history will guide further investigations and avoid unnecessary testing.

50 Per rectum bleeding

Definition: Bleeding from the rectum.

Differentials

- *Upper gastrointestinal (GI) tract*: see Chapter 37
- *GI tract* (blood will be mixed in with stool – haematochezia): inflammatory bowel disease (IBD), malignancy, diverticular disease
- *Lower GI tract* (fresh PR bleeding): diverticular disease, IBD (proctitis), infective diarrhoea, lymphogranuloma venereum (chlamydial) proctitis
- *Perianal disease* (blood usually separate from stool): anal fissures, fistula in ano, haemorrhoids, perianal herpes simplex virus/human papillomavirus/ syphilis

History

History of presenting complaint
- Description of bleed
- Type of blood seen
  - Fresh, bright red
  - Dark blood
  - Clots
  - Black sticky stool
- Seen where
  - Mixed in with stool
  - In the pan
  - On wiping only
- Amount of blood

Medical Student Survival Skills: History Taking and Communication Skills, First Edition.
Philip Jevon and Steve Odogwu.
© 2020 John Wiley & Sons Ltd. Published 2020 by John Wiley & Sons Ltd.
Companion website: www.wiley.com/go/jevon/medicalstudent

- Number of episodes of bleeding
- Normal frequency of bowel movements
  - Any recent change in bowel habit
- Normal consistency of stool
- Associated symptoms
  - Painful defecation
  - Constipation/diarrhoea
  - Abdominal pain
  - Nausea/vomiting
- Systems review
  - Weight loss
  - Fatigue
  - Night sweats
- Symptoms of significant blood loss
  - Chest pain
  - Palpitations
  - Shortness of breath
  - Lightheadedness/postural hypotension

Past medical history
- Inflammatory bowel disease
- Constipation
- Arthritis/psoriasis
- Previous malignancies

Drug history
- Current medications
- Allergies

Social history
- Smoker
- Low fibre diet
- Reduced exercise
- Sexual history
- Travel history

Family history
- Bowel cancer

OSCE Key Learning Points

✔ Do not forget to ask about red flag symptoms – any recent change in bowel habit and weight loss

 NB Any change in bowel habit, especially in the elderly, should be fully investigated.

51 Preoperative assessment

Definition: An assessment of the patient before (elective) surgery to determine their fitness for the given procedure, as well as to determine the most suitable anaesthetic option.

History

The history should revolve around the patient's general medical health, history of the current illness, and previous anaesthetics. The history of the current illness is important, for example those undergoing orthopaedic surgery for a fractured neck of the femur may be doing so as a result of a simple mechanical fall or as a result of more sinister pathology (e.g. cardiogenic syncope, following a cerebrovascular accident [CVA] or epileptic seizure, bony metastases or primary cancer). The history should be focused around the following points.

- Age
- Present illness requiring surgery and *cause*
- Recent general health
- Cardiovascular system and reserve
  - Especially ischaemic heart disease (myocardial infarction/angina) and heart failure
  - Uncontrolled hypertension
  - Especially peripheral vascular disease
  - Uncontrolled hypertension
  - Any history of anticoagulation
- Respiratory system and reserve
  - Especially chronic obstructive pulmonary disease (COPD), bronchiectasis, and chronic bronchitis
  - An objective assessment of aerobic fitness, e.g. exercise tolerance in metres

Medical Student Survival Skills: History Taking and Communication Skills, First Edition.
Philip Jevon and Steve Odogwu.
© 2020 John Wiley & Sons Ltd. Published 2020 by John Wiley & Sons Ltd.
Companion website: www.wiley.com/go/jevon/medicalstudent

- Renal function
  - Especially any degree of chronic kidney disease
- Neurology
  - Especially any history of CVA or transient ischaemic attack (TIA) and their residual effects
- Endocrine system
  - Especially any history of diabetes
- Gastrointestinal system
  - Especially pertaining to reflux and hiatus hernia
- Social history
  - Especially smoking and alcohol history
- Current medications
  - Including recently started, stopped, or new medications
  - Especially medications instructed to be withheld before surgery, e.g. angiotensin converting enzyme inhibitors
- Allergies
- History of prior operations and anaesthetics
  - Difficult intubation
  - Malignant hyperpyrexia, pseudocholinesterase deficiency

An assessment of the airway should then follow.

52 Per vaginum bleeding in pregnancy

Definition: Vaginal bleeding during pregnancy.

Differentials

- *Common*: early – miscarriage, ectopic pregnancy; late – placenta praevia, placental abruption, onset of labour
- *Rare*: early – molar pregnancy; late – vasa praevia; throughout – non-uterine bleeding (cervical, vaginal, etc.)

History

 NB Assess for hypovolaemic shock (obstetric emergency!).

History of presenting complaint
- Volume of bleeding (including any clots and products of conception)
- Duration and frequency
- Any related abdominal pain
- Preceding factors (trauma, intercourse)
- Foetal movements (if > 20 weeks)
- Other PV fluid loss
- Previous bleeding in this pregnancy
- Last menstrual period (LMP) and gestation
- Dating/20 week ultrasound scan results
- Position of placenta
- Rhesus status/blood group

Medical Student Survival Skills: History Taking and Communication Skills, First Edition.
Philip Jevon and Steve Odogwu.
© 2020 John Wiley & Sons Ltd. Published 2020 by John Wiley & Sons Ltd.
Companion website: www.wiley.com/go/jevon/medicalstudent

Past medical and obstetric history
- Explore all previous pregnancies including miscarriages, terminations, and still births
- Previous deliveries: mode of delivery, gestations, complications (during and afterwards)
- Past gynaecological history, including cervical sampling ('smear test') results
- Other medical problems, especially clotting disorders
- Hereditary disorders

Past surgical history
- Previous uterine surgery, including caesarean section
- Gynaecological or abdominal surgeries

Medications and allergies
- Current medications
- Medications used at any time in this pregnancy
- Over the counter medications, including use of folic acid
- Allergies

Social history
- Current partner(s) and family support
- Smoking, alcohol, and illicit drug use

OSCE Key Learning Points

✔ In particular, remember to ask about previous pregnancies and whether any complications occurred

 NB Rhesus negative women with bleeding during pregnancy may require anti-D injection to prevent rhesus D alloimmunisation.

 Uncommon presentations

Placental abruption may present only with abdominal pain and no bleeding.

 Common misinterpretations and pitfalls

Bleeding from the urethra, anus, or skin may be misinterpreted as vaginal bleeding.

53 Pruritus

Definition: Itching of the skin.

Differentials

- *Common*: eczema, urticaria, psoriasis
- *Rare*: malignancy (e.g. lymphoma), polycythaemia rubra vera, psychosis

History

History of presenting complaint
- Site – where did it start, has it spread to anywhere else
- Onset, triggers (e.g. animal hair, grass, food, detergents or soap, new medications)
- Exacerbating factors (e.g. night time for scabies, after baths for polycythaemia rubra vera)
- Associated rash or bleeding
- Any household contacts affected
- Any weight loss, anorexia, lethargy, fever, lumps/bumps, jaundice (including pale stools, dark urine)

Past medical history
- Previous skin disease
- History of atopy (asthma, hay fever)
- Liver disease, inflammatory bowel disease, coeliac disease, diabetes mellitus, thyroid disease
- Any other illnesses
- Could the patient be pregnant

Medical Student Survival Skills: History Taking and Communication Skills, First Edition.
Philip Jevon and Steve Odogwu.
© 2020 John Wiley & Sons Ltd. Published 2020 by John Wiley & Sons Ltd.
Companion website: www.wiley.com/go/jevon/medicalstudent

Medications and allergies
- Current medications; any new drugs, oral contraceptives
- Allergies

Family history
- Any family members with similar symptoms
- Any illnesses that run in the family

Social history
- Who patient lives with
- Occupation (e.g. healthcare setting) – related to rash?
- Smoking and alcohol
- Recent foreign travel

OSCE Key Learning Points

✔ If patient has systemic symptoms, use a focused systems review to find out the underlying medical condition

 NB Pruritus may be a symptom of malignancy!

 NB Ask to examine the skin as well as other systems, especially for lymphadenopathy and hepatosplenomegaly.

 Common misinterpretations and pitfalls

Pruritus is a non-specific symptom but can have underlying medical conditions (e.g. pruritus can precede jaundice by months or years in primary biliary cirrhosis).

54 Pervaginal bleed

Definition: A pervaginal bleed is any bleed from the vagina including the vaginal wall.

Differentials

- *Younger patient*: menstruation, miscarriage, cervical cancer, trauma, fibroids, ectropion
- *Older patient*: cancer (ovarian, endometrial), fibroids, polyps, atrophic changes

History

History of presenting complaint
- Onset, frequency.
- Quantify – pads/hour
- Clots – size (the size of a 50p coin or your palm?)
- Associated abdominal pain or bloating – use the SOCRATES approach (see Chapter 8)
- Inter-menstrual bleeding, post-coital bleeding, post-menopausal bleeding
- Any weight loss

Obstetric and gynaecological history
- Last smear
- Gravidity, pariety including type of delivery and any terminations or miscarriages
- Last menstrual period, regularity of periods
- Contraception, hormone replacement therapy
- Age of menses, menopause

Medical Student Survival Skills: History Taking and Communication Skills, First Edition.
Philip Jevon and Steve Odogwu.
© 2020 John Wiley & Sons Ltd. Published 2020 by John Wiley & Sons Ltd.
Companion website: www.wiley.com/go/jevon/medicalstudent

Past medical and surgical history
- Any abdominal operations
- Any other illness; establish if there are normal urinary and bowel habits
- Any bleeding/haematological history

Medications and allergies
- Allergies
- Any anticoagulant or non-steroidal anti-inflammatory drug use

Family history
- Ovarian, endometrial, breast, or colon cancer

OSCE Key Learning Points

✔ More serious causes should be excluded before assuming the cause is benign
✔ Do not forget to ask if the patient is pregnant!

 Common misinterpretations and pitfalls

Haematuria and bleeding from the rectum can sometimes be misinterpreted as PV bleeding, so beware!

 NB Always examine the abdomen, do a vaginal examination and speculum examination, and exclude anaemia.

(55) Pervaginal discharge

Definition: Discharge from the vagina which is different to normal.

Differentials

- *Common*: normal physiological discharge, thrush, bacterial vaginosis, chlamydia, gonorrhoea, pelvic inflammatory disease, atrophic vaginitis in postmenopausal women
- *Rare*: trichomoniasis, foreign body, genital tract malignancy, fistulae, cervical polyp, allergic reaction

History

 NB This can be an embarrassing topic for some patients. It is important to put the patient at ease and use simple terms so they understand.

History of presenting complaint
- Duration and onset of symptoms
- Nature of discharge – colour and consistency – what has changed from normal
- Does the discharge smell offensive
- Any itching or soreness
- Any rash
- Any dysuria
- Any dyspareunia – superficial or deep
- Any abnormal bleeding – intermenstrual, post-coital, post-menopausal

Medical Student Survival Skills: History Taking and Communication Skills, First Edition.
Philip Jevon and Steve Odogwu.
© 2020 John Wiley & Sons Ltd. Published 2020 by John Wiley & Sons Ltd.
Companion website: www.wiley.com/go/jevon/medicalstudent

- Any pelvic pain
- Any abdominal pain – use the SOCRATES approach (see Chapter 8)
- Any fevers or feeling generally unwell
- Sexually active at present
- Take brief sexual history – see Chapter 60
- Any chance patient could be pregnant at the moment
- Any history of trauma
- Any history of possible foreign body or cause of allergy

Past medical and surgical history
- Contraception history – what has been taken in past, what currently on
- Menstrual history – menarche, length of cycle, duration of typical period, regularity, heaviness or pain, age of menopause if post-menopausal
- Smear history – whether had smears, any abnormal smears, whether up to date
- Any medical conditions including diabetes, immunodeficiency, recurrent urinary tract infections
- Any operations – especially gynaecological
- Obstetric history
  - Number of previous pregnancies including miscarriages, terminations, and still births
  - Number of live births – gestation, mode of delivery, any problems

Medications and allergies
- Any regular medications, any steroids, or recent antibiotic courses
- Any allergies

Family history
- Any family history of any gynaecological malignancy

Social history
- Who lives at home
- Occupation
- Smoking – number per day and for how many years
- Alcohol – number of units per week

OSCE Key Learning Points

✔ It is important to take a full sexual and gynaecological history and a brief obstetric history in order to better inform your diagnosis

✔ Red flag symptoms are deep dyspareunia, inter-menstrual or post-coital bleeding, and pelvic pain

 Common misinterpretations and pitfalls

Although infection is a common cause of vaginal discharge, it is important to consider other causes particularly in older patients.

 NB Be aware of safeguarding issues. If sexually active, are they over 16 years old? Is there any possibility of domestic or sexual abuse?

56 Rash

Definition: Change in the appearance or texture of the skin.

Differentials

- *Infections*:
  - Bacterial – meningococcal septicaemia (rare, life-threatening), cellulitis, impetigo
  - Viral – chickenpox (varicella zoster virus), shingles (herpes zoster), cold sore/genital herpes (herpes simplex), viral exanthema
  - Fungal – Candida, tinea capitis/corporis/pedis
  - Parasites – scabies, lice
- *Acute*: Stevens–Johnson syndrome (rare, life-threatening), erythema nodosum, urticaria, contact dermatitis
- *Chronic*: eczema, psoriasis
- *Systemic*: vasculitis (e.g. systemic lupus erythematosus [SLE]), arthropathies (e.g. rheumatoid arthritis), diabetes mellitus, thyroid disorders, human immunodeficiency virus

History

History of presenting complaint
- Obtain description of appearance – colour, texture
- Site – where did it start, where did it spread to
- Onset, triggers (e.g. animal hair, grass, food, detergents or soap, trauma, new medications)
- Associated features: itch, bleeding, discharge
- Any household contacts affected
- Any weight loss, fever, joint pain, swelling
- How is the rash affecting you

Medical Student Survival Skills: History Taking and Communication Skills, First Edition.
Philip Jevon and Steve Odogwu.
© 2020 John Wiley & Sons Ltd. Published 2020 by John Wiley & Sons Ltd.
Companion website: www.wiley.com/go/jevon/medicalstudent

Past medical history
- Previous skin disease
- History of atopy (asthma, hay fever)
- Inflammatory bowel disease, coeliac disease, rheumatoid arthritis, SLE, diabetes, thyroid disease
- Any other illnesses

Medications and allergies
- Current medications; any new drugs (especially recent antibiotics), oral contraceptives
- Allergies – what reaction

Family history
- Any family members with similar symptoms
- Any illnesses that run in the family

Social history
- Who patient lives with
- Occupation (e.g. healthcare setting) – related to rash?
- Smoking and alcohol
- Recent foreign travel

OSCE Key Learning Points

✔ Focus on triggers (especially a thorough drug history) and whether it is contagious

✔ Explore the psychological effects on the patient (e.g. low mood, poor self-esteem)

 NB Do not forget to ask about systemic symptoms such as weight loss, fever, and joint pain for an underlying systemic diagnosis.

(57) Red eye – painless

Definition: An eye that presents with localised or generalised redness, secondary to injection, prominence, or rupture of the scleral or conjunctival vasculature.

Differentials

- *Immediate referral*: endophthalmitis (rarely presents without pain), chemical eye injury (normally causes pain/soreness)
- *24 hour referral*: foreign body (does not always cause pain)
- *Routine referral*: eyelid abnormalities (entropion, ectropion), trichiasis (ingrowing eyelashes), pterygium
- *No need for ophthalmic referral unless not resolving or red flag symptoms*: episcleritis, conjunctivitis (normally cause soreness/pain), blepharitis, chalazion, subconjunctival haemorrhage, keratoconjunctivitis sicca (dry eye)

NB Subconjunctival haemorrhage should be referred for further medical investigation within 24 hours if the patient is on anticoagulation drugs or has a very high blood pressure.

History

History of presenting complaint
- Important to ask from the beginning whether the vision has been affected
- Important to ask from the beginning whether the patient has any known ocular pathology or past history
- The onset of redness – was it sudden or gradual, what was the patient doing at the time (in particular was there any trauma)
- How long have the symptoms been going on for

Medical Student Survival Skills: History Taking and Communication Skills, First Edition.
Philip Jevon and Steve Odogwu.
© 2020 John Wiley & Sons Ltd. Published 2020 by John Wiley & Sons Ltd.
Companion website: www.wiley.com/go/jevon/medicalstudent

165

- Has it worsened or improved
- Is this the first such episode
- Has there been any pain or soreness
- If the vision has deteriorated, ascertain the context of this – sudden/gradual, improved/worsened, central/peripheral, complete/partial
- Associated ocular symptoms
  - Discharge
  - Gritty sensation
  - Lacrimation
  - Photophobia
  - Haloes around lights
  - Diplopia
- Systemic symptoms
  - Fever
  - Cough
  - Coryza (especially purulent rhinorrhoea)
  - Rashes
  - Diarrhoea and/or vomiting
  - Headaches
  - Meningism
  - Arthralgia
  - Urethral discharge (ask about sexual history)
- Does the patient wear contact lenses – if so monthly or daily disposables; ascertain their level of hygiene and correct use (e.g. over wear)
- Any recent ocular surgery

Past medical history
- Known ocular disease
- Hypertension
- Diabetes
- Previous infection – tuberculosis, syphilis, herpes
- Previous sinusitis
- Systemic disease
  - Rheumatoid arthritis
  - Ankylosing spondylitis
  - Inflammatory bowel disease
  - Psoriatic arthritis
  - Sarcoidosis

Medications
- Drug allergies
- Known eye drops
- Anticoagulants
- Antiplatelets

Social history
- Smoking
- Alcohol
- Recreational drug use (IV drug use)
- Occupation

OSCE Key Learning Points

✔ A painless red eye usually does not require immediate ophthalmology referral

✔ A detailed history and examination is vital in reaching the correct diagnosis or at least a small number of differentials

Red flag symptoms
- Reduced visual acuity – anything obstructing the visual axis and could be corneal pathology or optic disc involvement
- Photophobia – can indicate corneal oedema, corneal abrasion, excessive light entering the eye due to iris abnormalities (unable to constrict), or be associated with meningeal irritation
- Pain in the eye
- Irregular appearance or function of pupil

NB
- If the symptoms are not resolving or indeed worsening, it warrants ophthalmic referral
- Painless red eye can progress into a painful red eye if not managed accurately

 Common misinterpretations and pitfalls

Blurred vision that clears with blinking is not a deterioration of vision.

58 Red eye – painful

Definition: A painful eye that presents with localised or generalised redness, secondary to injection, prominence, or rupture of the scleral or conjunctival vasculature.

Differentials

- *Immediate referral*: endophthalmitis, acute angle closure glaucoma, trauma to the globe, chemical eye injury (especially alkali burns), bacterial keratitis with hypopyon (white blood cells in anterior chamber), orbital cellulitis, corneal ulceration
- *24 hour referral*: scleritis, anterior uveitis, keratitis, corneal foreign body
- *No need for ophthalmic referral unless not resolving or red flag symptoms*: episcleritis, conjunctivitis, blepharitis, dry eye

 NB Conditions causing painful red eye typically affect the anterior segment.

History

History of presenting complaint
- Important to ask from the beginning whether the vision has been affected
- Important to ask from the beginning whether the patient has any known ocular pathology or past history
- Onset of pain and redness – did they coincide, was it sudden or gradual, what was the patient doing at the time (in particular was there any trauma)
- How long have the symptoms been going on for
- Has it worsened or improved

Medical Student Survival Skills: History Taking and Communication Skills, First Edition.
Philip Jevon and Steve Odogwu.
© 2020 John Wiley & Sons Ltd. Published 2020 by John Wiley & Sons Ltd.
Companion website: www.wiley.com/go/jevon/medicalstudent

- Is this the first such episode
- Describe the pain – site, character, radiation, timing, exacerbating and alleviating factors, severity
- If the vision has deteriorated, ascertain the context of this – sudden/gradual, improved/worsened, central/peripheral, complete/partial
- Associated ocular symptoms
  - Discharge
  - Gritty sensation
  - Lacrimation
  - Photophobia
  - Haloes around lights
  - Diplopia
- Systemic symptoms
  - Fever
  - Cough
  - Coryza (especially purulent rhinorrhoea)
  - Rashes
  - Diarrhoea and/or vomiting
  - Headaches
  - Meningism
  - Arthralgia
  - Urethral discharge (ask about sexual history)
- Does the patient wear contact lenses – if so monthly or daily disposables: ascertain their level of hygiene and correct use (e.g. over wear)
- Any recent ocular surgery

Past medical history
- Known ocular disease
- Hypertension
- Diabetes
- Previous infection – tuberculosis, syphilis, herpes
- Previous sinusitis
- Systemic disease
  - Rheumatoid arthritis
  - Ankylosing spondylitis
  - Inflammatory bowel disease
  - Psoriatic arthritis
  - Sarcoidosis

Medications and allergies
- Drug allergies
- Known eye drops

Social history
- Smoking
- Alcohol
- Recreational drug use (IV drug use)
- Occupation

OSCE Key Learning Points

✔ A painful red eye may not always require immediate ophthalmology referral
✔ A detailed history and examination is vital in reaching the correct diagnosis or at least a small number of differentials

Red flag symptoms
- Reduced visual acuity – anything obstructing the visual axis and could be corneal pathology or optic disc involvement
- Photophobia – can indicate corneal oedema, corneal abrasion, excessive light entering the eye due to iris abnormalities (unable to constrict), or be associated with meningeal irritation
- Pain in the eye
- Irregular appearance or function of pupil

NB
- An acute abdomen and red eye in the elderly can be an indication of acute angle closure glaucoma
- Increased pain in the eye when reading may indicate an anterior uveitis (iris constricting)
- Proptosis or diplopia is an indicator of orbital involvement (such as orbital cellulitis)
- Corneal transplant and a painful red eye is a sign of graft rejection

⚠ Common misinterpretations and pitfalls

- Blurred vision that clears with blinking is not a deterioration of vision
- Scleritis can present in the elderly without redness
- Endophthalmitis can present without pain

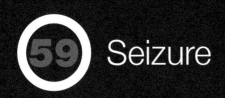

59 Seizure

Definition: Physical signs and symptoms due to uncontrolled abnormal electrical activity of the brain.

Types of Seizure

- *Focal/partial seizures* involve a localised part of the brain
  - Simple – intact consciousness
  - Complex – impaired consciousness
- *Generalised seizures* involve the entire brain
  - Tonic-clonic – stiffness followed by jerking movements, often preceded by an aura
  - Absence – sudden impairment of consciousness which is unresponsive to stimuli
  - Atonic – sudden loss of muscle tone (drop attacks)
  - Myoclonic – isolated jerking movement

Differentials

- *Common*: epilepsy, head trauma, metabolic disturbances (hypoglycaemia, hypocalcaemia, hyponatraemia, uraemia)
- *Rare*: raised intracranial pressure (tumour, abscess, cerebral oedema, aneurysm)

History

 NB It is important to obtain a collateral history from a witness.

Medical Student Survival Skills: History Taking and Communication Skills, First Edition.
Philip Jevon and Steve Odogwu.
© 2020 John Wiley & Sons Ltd. Published 2020 by John Wiley & Sons Ltd.
Companion website: www.wiley.com/go/jevon/medicalstudent

History of presenting complaint
- Any warning signs before the seizure
    - Visual changes – loss of vision, bright lights, floaters
    - Auditory changes – tinnitus, hallucinations
    - Prodrome – change in behaviour/mood, hours/days before the attack
- In what circumstance did the attack occur – flickering lights, alcohol intoxication
- Loss of consciousness
- Trauma involved
- Abnormal movement
    - Stiffness of muscles (tonic)
    - Twitching of muscles (clonic)
    - Remains still and stares blankly, unresponsive to external stimuli (absence)
- Loss of continence
- Change in colour – cyanotic, pale
- Tongue biting, drooling, grunting
- Duration of seizure
- After the seizure
    - Amnesia
    - Nausea or vomiting – typically associated with head injury
    - Confused/sleepy – typical after epileptic seizure
    - Aching muscles – typically after tonic-clonic seizure
- Is this the first attack
- Are the attacks becoming more frequent

Past medical and surgical history
- Diabetes, renal failure, metabolic disturbance
- Cerebral tumour, central nervous system infections – leading to raised intracranial pressure
- Any other illnesses
- Any previous surgery – especially neurological

Medications and allergies
- Current medications
- Allergies

Family history
- Any family members with similar episodes
- Any illnesses run in the family – especially epilepsy (strong genetic link)

Social history
- Smoking and alcohol
- IV drug use
- Who does the patient live with, any dependents

OSCE Key Learning Points

✔ Remember to ask about before the seizure, during the seizure, and after the seizure

 NB Sleep deprivation, alcohol intoxication/withdrawal, and infection are triggers of seizures.

⚠ Common misinterpretations and pitfalls

Because a patient has a seizure, this does not mean they have epilepsy. Epilepsy can only be diagnosed after two seizures within 2 years.

60 Sexual history from a female patient

OSCE Key Learning Points

✔ Be tactful, non-judgemental, and explain why you are asking these personal questions

History

History of presenting complaint
- Allow them to describe the problem or situation
  - Any symptoms, any concerns, recent contact, a check-up wanted
- Check for specific symptoms and risk of pregnancy
  - Vulval soreness or itch, ulcers, rashes, discharge (consistency, smell), dysuria, dyspareunia, last menstrual period (LMP), missed period, flu-like symptoms, jaundiced, etc.
- Discuss recent sexual contact
  - Obtain details for all partners at least in the last 3 months including time of contact, partner gender, partner symptoms, duration of relationship (boyfriend, one off), type of contact (oral, vaginal, anal), condom and contraception use
- Discuss risk of blood-borne virus transmission – human immunodeficiency virus (HIV), hepatitis B or C
  - Sexual contact with a partner from high risk area or known to have HIV, paid for or been paid for sex, injecting drugs, blood transfusion or surgery abroad, contact with MSM (men who have sex with men)
  - Antenatal or previous HIV testing

Medical Student Survival Skills: History Taking and Communication Skills, First Edition.
Philip Jevon and Steve Odogwu.
© 2020 John Wiley & Sons Ltd. Published 2020 by John Wiley & Sons Ltd.
Companion website: www.wiley.com/go/jevon/medicalstudent

Past medical and surgical history
- Previous sexually transmitted infections (STIs) and treatment
- Other medical/surgical problems

Gynaecological history
- LMP, cycle length and duration – any concerns
- Pregnancies, terminations, and miscarriages
- Contraception – use, compliance (missed pills, expired depot injection or implant)
- Cervical smear – up to date, abnormalities

Medications and allergies
- Especially antibiotics and enzyme-inducing medications that interact with oral contraceptives
- Allergies

Social history
- Smoking, alcohol, other illicit drugs

OSCE Key Learning Points

Sexual history taking: the five 'P's
- ✔ **P**artners
- ✔ **P**ractices
- ✔ **P**rotection from sexually transmitted diseases (STDs)
- ✔ **P**ast history of STDs
- ✔ **P**revention of pregnancy

61 Sexual history from a male patient

OSCE Key Learning Points

✔ Be tactful, non-judgemental, and explain why you are asking these personal questions

History

History of presenting complaint
- Allow them to describe the problem or situation
  - Any symptoms, any concerns, recent contact, a check-up wanted
- Check for specific symptoms
  - Penis soreness or itch, ulcers, rashes, discharge (consistency, smell), dysuria, dyspareunia, flu-like symptoms, jaundiced, etc.
- Discuss recent sexual contact
  - Obtain details for all partners at least in the last 3 months including time of contact, partner gender, partner symptoms, duration of relationship (girlfriend, one off), type of contact (oral, penis, anal), and condom use
- Discuss risk of blood-borne virus transmission – human immunodeficiency virus (HIV), hepatitis B or C
  - Sexual contact with a partner from high risk area or known to have HIV, paid for or been paid for sex, injecting drugs, blood transfusion or surgery abroad, contact with MSM (men who have sex with men)
  - Previous HIV testing

Past medical and surgical history
- Previous sexually transmitted infections (STIs) and treatment
- Other medical/surgical problems

Medical Student Survival Skills: History Taking and Communication Skills, First Edition.
Philip Jevon and Steve Odogwu.
© 2020 John Wiley & Sons Ltd. Published 2020 by John Wiley & Sons Ltd.
Companion website: www.wiley.com/go/jevon/medicalstudent

Medications and allergies
- Especially medications that can cause erectile dysfunction (e.g. antihypertensives) / medications to treat erectile dysfunction (e.g. sildenafil)
- Allergies

Social history
- Smoking, alcohol, other illicit drugs

OSCE Key Learning Points

Sexual history taking: the four 'P's
✔ **P**artners
✔ **P**ractices
✔ **P**rotection from sexually transmitted diseases (STDs)
✔ **P**ast history of STDs

62 Shortness of breath

Definition: An unpleasant sensation of uncomfortable, rapid, or difficult breathing.

Differentials

- *Common*: obesity, smoking, asthma, chronic obstructive pulmonary disease (COPD), pneumonia, anaemia, congestive cardia failure, inhaled foreign body, pneumothorax, pulmonary embolism, malignancy, pulmonary fibrosis
- *Rare*: sarcoid, fibrosing alveolitis, tuberculosis (TB)

History

History of presenting complaint
- Ask the patient to describe the actual sensation they experience
- When it started
- Any chest pain/tightness
- Constant shortness of breath (SOB) or does it come and go, any particular time it is worse
- Associated symptoms – wheeze, cough, sputum, peripheral oedema, or systemic symptoms (headache, myalgia, pyrexia, lethargy)
- What activities are they unable to do due to the SOB
- How far can they walk on flat ground before breathlessness comes on; has this got worse or stayed the same
- Paroxsymal nocturnal dyspnoea, how many pillows do they use at night
- Enquire about anxiety symptoms – tingling in fingers, feeling light headed when they are SOB

Medical Student Survival Skills: History Taking and Communication Skills, First Edition.
Philip Jevon and Steve Odogwu.
© 2020 John Wiley & Sons Ltd. Published 2020 by John Wiley & Sons Ltd.
Companion website: www.wiley.com/go/jevon/medicalstudent

- Have they noticed if the SOB is linked to or triggered by any activity or particular environment
- Any weight loss

Past medical history
- Asthma, hay fever, COPD, cardiac disease

Medications and allergies
- Current medications – any inhalers in particular
- Corticosteroids
- Angiotensin converting enzyme inhibitors
- Aspirin or non-steroidal anti-inflammatory drugs
- Allergies

Family history
- Lung disease
- Smokers in the family
- Atopy – asthma, eczema, hay fever

Social history
- Occupation – exposure to dusts/allergens
- Smoking – how much and for how long
- Recent foreign travel – TB prevalent areas
- Pets/birds
- Effect of SOB on daily life and job

OSCE Key Learning Points

✔ In particular, remember to ask about smoking as this is a major risk factor for both respiratory and cardiovascular disease

 NB Obesity is one of the major causes of breathlessness – do not forget to ask about life style!

 Common misinterpretations and pitfalls

Establish early how long they have had SOB and how quickly it developed. The differentials for sudden dyspnoea are very different to dyspnoea developing over months.

63 Stridor

Definition: Loud, harsh, high pitched respiratory sound.

Cause

- *Inspiratory*: partial upper airway obstruction, usually extrathoracic
- *Expiratory*: complete airway obstruction, usually intrathoracic

Differentials

- *Acute*: inhaled foreign body, anaphylactic reaction, epiglottitis, croup (laryngotracheobronchitis), laryngitis, laryngospasm secondary to smoke inhalation
- *Chronic*: laryngomalacia, tumour (laryngeal, mediastinal), thyroid

History

History of presenting complaint
- Onset
- Severity – cyanosis, respiratory effort
- Positional
- Ingestion of substances
- Preceding illnesses
- Other symptoms – cough, chest pain, salivating
- Weight loss

Past medical history
- Respiratory illnesses
- Trauma

Medical Student Survival Skills: History Taking and Communication Skills, First Edition.
Philip Jevon and Steve Odogwu.
© 2020 John Wiley & Sons Ltd. Published 2020 by John Wiley & Sons Ltd.
Companion website: www.wiley.com/go/jevon/medicalstudent

Medications and allergies
- For acute stridor you need to establish if the patient has recently ingested any new medications
- Allergies are paramount in this case, including non-medication allergies such as to seafood, wasps, etc.

Family history
- History of anaphylaxis

Social history
- Smoking, alcohol

OSCE Key Learning Points

✔ Stridor can be life-threatening
✔ Do not forget allergies!
✔ If you have established it is acute stridor, the first thing is *get help*! You will need an anaesthetist, physician, and ENT surgeon at the very least

 NB Chronic stridor in adults can indicate underlying malignancy.

 Uncommon presentations

Psychogenic stridor in young females.

64 Substance misuse

> **Definition:** The excessive use of a substance, for example alcohol or a drug.

Substance dependence is when an individual persists in the use of alcohol or drugs regardless of the problems related to its use. Repeated use may result in tolerance and withdrawal symptoms if stopped. Substance misuse can involve the use of alcohol, benzodiazepines, amphetamines, opiates, MDMA (3,4-methylenedioxy-methamphetamine), cannabis, and solvents.

History

 NB Infection control measures, introduction, and consent.

History of presenting complaint
- Type of drug
- Route of administration
- Frequency and amount used
- Duration of drug use
- Any triggers/stressors
- Assess dependence
  - Tolerance
  - Withdrawal
  - Impaired control
  - Neglect of activities
  - Use despite harm
  - Compulsive use

Medical Student Survival Skills: History Taking and Communication Skills, First Edition.
Philip Jevon and Steve Odogwu.
© 2020 John Wiley & Sons Ltd. Published 2020 by John Wiley & Sons Ltd.
Companion website: www.wiley.com/go/jevon/medicalstudent

- Salience
- Reinstatement after abstinence
- How are the drugs paid for and how much money is spent
- Other substances used
- Find out the patient's insight, e.g. advantages and disadvantages of the drug, thoughts of cutting down
- Screen for depression

Past medical history
- Physical health problems, e.g. chronic conditions
- Any previous drug overdoses
- Previous drug use and detoxification attempts

Past psychiatric history
- Mental health problems, e.g. mood disorders

Medications and allergies
- Current medications
- Allergies

Family history
- Any illnesses run in the family, e.g. psychiatric disorder

Social history
- Establish who the patient lives with and how they are affected
- Impact of drug on patient's life
- Is there social support available
- Smoking and alcohol
- Financial and legal matters, e.g. court cases

Risk assessment
- Assess risk to self and others
- IV use/clean needles/needle sharing

OSCE Key Learning Points

✔ Do not forget to ask about mental illness as there is a strong relationship between the two
✔ Establish the social situation

65 Swollen legs and ankles

Oedema is the expansion of the interstitial space with excess water. It results when the balance of forces promoting water movement out of the bloodstream are stronger than those acting to keep it in. The commonest causes of oedema clinically involve changes to hydrostatic and oncotic pressures.

Differentials

- *Pitting oedema* (usually bilateral):
  - *Increased hydrostatic pressure:* heart failure, tricuspid and pulmonary valve disease (regurgitation or stenosis), renal failure, venous insufficiency, venous obstruction (e.g. pelvic mass, pregnancy, inferior vena cava obstruction), iatrogenic (calcium channel blockers, IV fluid overload), hypothyroidism, pregnancy
  - *Decreased oncotic pressure:* liver failure, protein-wasting nephropathy (can lead to nephrotic syndrome), malnutrition, malabsorption
- *Non-pitting oedema*: primary lymphoedema, deep vein thrombosis (usually unilateral), malignancy (lymphoma, secondary infiltration), infection (erysipelas – cellulitis with lymph vessel involvement, filiariasis), iatrogenic (lymph node excision, radiotherapy)

History

History of presenting complaint
The key to narrowing the differential diagnosis is to enquire about the onset of the oedema and its related symptoms.

- Onset
  - Acute – deep vein thrombosis (DVT), acute renal failure, iatrogenic fluid overload)

Medical Student Survival Skills: History Taking and Communication Skills, First Edition.
Philip Jevon and Steve Odogwu.
© 2020 John Wiley & Sons Ltd. Published 2020 by John Wiley & Sons Ltd.
Companion website: www.wiley.com/go/jevon/medicalstudent

- – Subacute – infection, lymph node excision, hypothyroidism
- – Gradual – malignancy, heart/renal/liver failure, malnutrition, radiotherapy
- Associated symptoms
  - – Breathlessness, orthopnoea, chest pain (heart failure)
  - – Malaise, fatigue, itching, abdominal aching (renal failure)
  - – Jaundice, abdominal swelling, ataxia, encephalopathy (liver failure)
  - – Weight loss, fever, night sweats, abnormal lumps (malignancy, infection)
  - – Varicose veins, venous eczema, leg ulceration (venous insufficiency)

Past medical and surgical history
- Angina and myocardial infarction, valve replacements, rheumatic fever (heart disease)
- Diabetes, cystic kidneys, renal stones, benign prostatic hypertrophy (chronic renal failure)
- Autoimmune conditions, streptococcal infections, pelvic surgery (acute renal failure)
- Inflammatory bowel disease, coeliac disease, bowel resection, cystic fibrosis, chronic pancreatitis (malabsorption/malnutrition)
- Previous varicose veins, foot/ankle ulcers, DVT (chronic venous insufficiency)

Medications and allergies
- Calcium channel blockers (vasodilatory)
- Non-steroidal anti-inflammatory drugs, aminoglycosides, IV iodinated contrast, metformin, platinum compounds (acute renal failure)
- IV fluids (iatrogenic fluid overload)
- Allergies

Social history
- Smoking (heart disease, malignancy)
- Alcohol (liver failure)
- Travel history (infection, DVT, chronic hepatitis)

OSCE Key Learning Points

✔ Define the onset of oedema and related symptoms
✔ Aim to differentiate between cardiovascular causes and those associated with fluid overload and low protein states

Common misinterpretations and pitfalls

Swelling due to prolonged sitting is called 'dependent odema', and is not always abnormal. Always look for the level of the jugular venous pressure and complete a full cardiovascular examination.

66 Syncope

Definition: Transient loss of consciousness due to decreased perfusion to the brain, which is characterised by a rapid onset, and a spontaneous complete recovery.

Synonyms for syncope include passing out, blackout, and fainting.

Differentials

- *Common:*
  - Neurologically related – vasovagal syncope, situational syncope
  - Hypovolaemia
  - Iatrogenic – antihypertensives
  - Cardiac related – arrhythmias, valvular lesions, hypertrophic obstructive cardiomyopathy
  - Orthostatic hypotension (postural hypotension)
- *Rare*: carotid sinus hypersensitivity, Brugada's syndrome, Addison's disease

History

 NB It is important to obtain a collateral history from a witness.

History of presenting complaint
- Any warning signs before the syncope
  - Nausea
  - Sweating

Medical Student Survival Skills: History Taking and Communication Skills, First Edition.
Philip Jevon and Steve Odogwu.
© 2020 John Wiley & Sons Ltd. Published 2020 by John Wiley & Sons Ltd.
Companion website: www.wiley.com/go/jevon/medicalstudent

- – Decreased visual fields
- – Lightheadedness
- – Dizziness
- – Weakness
- – Blurred vision
- In what circumstance did the attack occur
  - – Standing up from sitting – orthostatic hypotension
  - – Strong emotion/fear/prolonged standing – vasovagal syncope
  - – Did it occur during a cough/sneeze, defecation, or micturition – situational syncope
- Loss of consciousness, if so, for how long
- Any palpitations
- Loss of continence (may occur in vasovagal syncope)
- Abnormal movement during syncope
  - – Twitching of muscles (clonic) – may be a feature of syncope
- Change in colour – cyanotic, pale
- After the syncope
  - – How long did it take to fully recover
  - – Confused/amnesia/sleepiness
- Is this the first attack
- Are the attacks becoming more frequent

Past medical and surgical history
- Arrhythmias – atrial fibrillation, supraventricular or ventricular tachycardia, prolonged QT syndrome, heart block
- Valvular lesions – aortic regurgitation, aortic stenosis
- Diabetes (autonomic neuropathy)
- Addison's disease
- Any other illnesses
- Any previous surgery

Medications and allergies
- Current medications – beta-blockers, angiotensin converting enzyme inhibitors, diuretics, calcium channel blockers (may cause excessive hypotension)
- Allergies

Family history
- Any family members with similar episodes
- Any illnesses run in the family – arrhythmias, hypertrophic obstructive cardiomyopathy

Social history
- Smoking and alcohol
- Who does the patient live with, any dependents

OSCE Key Learning Points

✔ Remember to ask about before the syncope, during the syncope, and after the syncope

 NB Cardiac-related syncope typically occurs without warning, lasts for only seconds, and has a fast recovery with no confusion/amnesia.

 NB Twitching (clonic activity) during loss of consciousness may occur in syncope. It does not always mean it is a seizure. However, stiffness (tonic activity) does not occur in syncope, only in seizures.

 Common misinterpretations and pitfalls

The causes of syncope exclude seizures, coma, and shock but these may form part of the differential diagnosis.

67 Tiredness/lethargy

Definition: The state of being weary or fatigued.

Differentials

- *Common*: simple physiological tiredness, depression, anaemia, during or after infection
- *Rare*: chronic fatigue syndrome, heart failure, malignancy, hypothyroidism

History

NB Red flag symptoms: see Table 67.1.

History of presenting complaint
- When it started
- Duration
- Continuous or worse at a particular time of the day
- First episode (if not, what previous investigations has the patient had)
- History of recent infection
- Is patient aware of any potential associated factors, e.g. new baby, working longer hours
- Sleep pattern
- Associated symptoms, e.g. change in bowel habit including PR bleeding
- Muscle weakness
- Mood, apathy, difficulty in concentration, early morning waking (depression)
- Weight loss, appetite, changes in diet (e.g. vegetarian)

Medical Student Survival Skills: History Taking and Communication Skills, First Edition.
Philip Jevon and Steve Odogwu.
© 2020 John Wiley & Sons Ltd. Published 2020 by John Wiley & Sons Ltd.
Companion website: www.wiley.com/go/jevon/medicalstudent

Table 67.1 More common red flag/warning symptoms

System	Red flag symptoms	Associated conditions
Cardiovascular	Increasing breathlessness	Heart failure
Respiratory	Haemoptysis, night sweats, cough Increasing breathlessness	Tuberculosis Bronchial carcinoma (may also have haemoptysis)
	Daytime somnolence	Obstructive sleep apnoea
Gastrointestinal	Change in bowel habit, weight loss, anorexia	Colorectal carcinoma Malabsorption Inflammatory bowel disease
Endocrine	Weight gain/cold intolerance	Hypothyroidism
Haematological	Pallor Easy bruising Night sweats	Iron deficiency anaemia Leukaemia Lymphoma
Neurological	Muscle weakness	Myasthenia gravis Myopathies Motor neuron disease

Past medical and surgical history
- History of chronic disease, e.g. ischaemic heart disease, iron deficiency anaemia, malignancy
- History of depression, anxiety
- Surgical history

Medications and allergies
- Current medications
- Benzodiazepines, antidepressants, herbal medications
- Compliance
- Allergies

Family history
- History of malignancy
- History of chronic fatigue syndrome

Social history
- Employment status – if employed, is work stimulating the patient
- Relationship status
- Any dependents, e.g. children or elderly family
- Smoking, alcohol, illicit drug use (if appropriate)
- How is the tiredness affecting their daily life

OSCE Key Learning Points

- ✔ A systems review is a great tool to use with a non-specific symptom like tiredness/lethargy. Especially when trying to identify or rule out accompanying red flag symptoms
- ✔ Chronic fatigue syndrome is a diagnosis of exclusion

 Common misinterpretations and pitfalls

Even if you identify a physiological cause of tiredness, e.g. lack of sleep, in an exam situation you must *also* rule out any medical/organic causes.

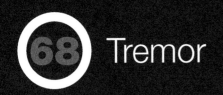

68 Tremor

Definition: A rhythmic oscillation of limbs, trunk, head, or tongue.

Differentials

- *Physiological*: anxiety, hyperthyroidism, effects of alcohol and drug use.
- *Neurological*: Parkinsonism, cerebellar disease, Wilson's disease, syphilis
- *Familial*: essential tremor (autosomal dominant)

History

History of presenting complaint
- Site affected, unilateral or bilateral
- Age of onset and progression
- Frequency – comes and goes or is constant
- Character – rapid or slow
- Present at rest
- Triggers – worse on movements, arms outstretched
- Relieving factors – alcohol
- Associated neurological symptoms, bradykinesia, rigidity, dementia
- Other cerebellar symptoms such as ataxia and speech disturbance
- History of weight loss, sweating

Past medical history
- Neurological history – anxiety, Parkinson's disease, epilepsy, dementia
- Any thyroid problems
- Asthma, chronic obstructive pulmonary disease

Medical Student Survival Skills: History Taking and Communication Skills, First Edition.
Philip Jevon and Steve Odogwu.
© 2020 John Wiley & Sons Ltd. Published 2020 by John Wiley & Sons Ltd.
Companion website: www.wiley.com/go/jevon/medicalstudent

Medications and allergies
- Current medications
- Beta-agonists
- Allergies

Social history
- Alcohol
- Illicit drug use

OSCE Key Learning Points

✔ In particular, ask about age of onset and triggers, e.g. worse at rest or on movement. This will help determine the underlying cause
✔ On examination look for cerebellar signs and Parkinsonism

 Common misinterpretations and pitfalls

Establish the exact character of the tremor symptoms and the site involved, and rule out symptoms of rigours, seizures, and myoclonic jerks.

69 Unilateral leg swelling

Definition: Increase in size of one leg.

Differentials

- *Common*: deep vein thrombosis (DVT), cellulitis, trauma, ruptured Baker's cyst
- *Rare*: abnormal lymphatic drainage (compression by mass, lymphoma, trypanosomiasis), Milroy's syndrome, Klippel–Trénaunay–Weber syndrome

History

NB Differentiate between unilateral and bilateral leg swelling.

History of presenting complaint
- Onset and duration of leg swelling
- Exacerbating and relieving factors, e.g. having legs up, walking, better in the morning
- Any skin changes, e.g. erythema/warmth, ulcers, eczema
- History of trauma, e.g. insect bite, wound, bruising
- Pain or tenderness: SOCRATES approach (see Chapter 8)
- Mobility: recent immobility, mobility affected
- Fever, feeling unwell generally, confusion
- Abdominal pain, weight loss, appetite loss, change in bowel habit, night sweats
- Any lumps/bumps in groin or abdomen
- Recent onset of shortness of breath

Medical Student Survival Skills: History Taking and Communication Skills, First Edition.
Philip Jevon and Steve Odogwu.
© 2020 John Wiley & Sons Ltd. Published 2020 by John Wiley & Sons Ltd.
Companion website: www.wiley.com/go/jevon/medicalstudent

- Varicose veins
- Recent travel
- History of arthritis

Past medical and surgical history
- History of DVT, pulmonary embolism (PE), or any thrombotic events
- History of recent surgery, hospitalisation, or cast
- History of malignancy/radiotherapy
- History of surgery on affected limb
- History of diabetes
- Pregnancy
- Any other medical/surgical problems

Medications and allergies
- Current medications: especially oral contraceptives and hormone replacement therapy
- Compliance with medications
- Allergy history

Family history
- DVT/PE
- Hereditary lymphatic disorders
- Any medical conditions running in the family

Social history
- Who patient lives with
- Current mobility and ability to do activities of daily living
- Current housing situation – bungalow/stairs
- Occupation history
- Smoking and passive smoking
- Recent travel
- Alcohol history and IV drug use

OSCE Key Learning Points

✔ Consider diabetes in anyone who presents with cellulitis – check bedside blood sugar
✔ Always do a Wells score for anyone you suspect may have DVT

NB Do not forget about pelvic malignancy as a cause for unilateral leg swelling; always examine the groin and abdomen.

 Common misinterpretations and pitfalls

- For a DVT:
  - If the Wells score is ≥ 2, do not do a D-dimer test if a Doppler scan is available within 4 hours
  - If the Wells score is ≤ 1, do a D-dimer test
  - If the D-dimer is raised and there is a negative Doppler, the patient needs to return for a repeat Doppler scan in 6–8 days
- Patients on anticoagulation can still get DVT

70 Varicose veins

Definition: Dilated, tortuous veins on the legs due to incompetence of the valves in the venous system.

History

History of presenting complaint
- Obtain description of varicose veins
- Onset, triggers
- Associated heaviness and pain on legs, paraesthesia
- Skin discoloration, ulcers
- History of oedema (onset, variation throughout the day)
- Risk factors (pregnancy, previous trauma, deep vein thrombosis [DVT], diabetes)
- Impact (how has this affected life)

Past medical and surgical history
- History of previous venous problems
- DVT, myocardial infarction, diabetes, thrombophilia
- Any other illness
- Previous surgery

Medications and allergies
- Medications, over the counter preparations
- Allergies

Family history
- Similar symptoms in family
- Inherited family disorders

Medical Student Survival Skills: History Taking and Communication Skills, First Edition.
Philip Jevon and Steve Odogwu.
© 2020 John Wiley & Sons Ltd. Published 2020 by John Wiley & Sons Ltd.
Companion website: www.wiley.com/go/jevon/medicalstudent

Social history
- Who patient lives with
- Smoking and alcohol
- Occupation

Communication skills
- Building rapport and listening
- Acknowledging patient concerns, responding appropriately

 NB Do not forget to ask about occupation.

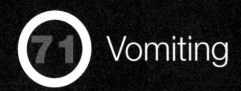 Vomiting

Definition: Forceful expulsion of stomach's contents.

Differentials

- *Common*: gastroenteritis (viral and bacterial), inflammatory lesion (ulcer or malignancy), drugs, bowel obstruction
- *Rare*: metabolic (e.g. uraemia, hyperglycaemia), neurogenic (raised intracranial pressure, vestibulocochlear disease)

History

 NB Infection control measures.

History of presenting complaint
- Duration of symptoms, onset, frequency, triggers (e.g. food or stress)
- Frequency – e.g. immediately after food or early morning
- Obtain description of vomit (solid food, liquid)
- Colour of vomit; content – coffee ground (digested blood) or fresh blood, faeculent, green (bile)
- Associated pain
- Abdominal pain – use SOCRATES template (see Chapter 8)
- Associated symptoms – diarrhoea, dysphagia, weight loss, fever, headache
- Any unusual food consumption

Medical Student Survival Skills: History Taking and Communication Skills, First Edition.
Philip Jevon and Steve Odogwu.
© 2020 John Wiley & Sons Ltd. Published 2020 by John Wiley & Sons Ltd.
Companion website: www.wiley.com/go/jevon/medicalstudent

Past medical and surgical history
- Constipation, diarrhoea, gastro-oesophageal reflux disease, ulcerative disease
- Any other illnesses
- Any previous surgery – especially abdominal

Medications and allergies
- Current medications, opiates, cytotoxics, antibiotics
- Allergies

Family history
- Any family members with similar symptoms
- Any illnesses that run in the family

Social history
- Who patient lives with
- Occupation (e.g. healthcare setting or around food)
- Smoking and alcohol
- Recent foreign travel

OSCE Key Learning Points

✔ In particular, remember to ask about weight loss and unusual food consumption

 NB Be aware of when public health bodies need to be informed.

 Common misinterpretations and pitfalls

Establish early a description of the vomit – vomiting up just-swallowed food is very different to coffee ground vomit.

72 Weight gain

Definition: Obesity is defined as a body mass index (BMI) of $>30\,kg\,m^{-2}$. Normal BMI is $18.5-24.9\,kg\,m^{-2}$; overweight is $25-30\,kg\,m^{-2}$.

Differentials

- *Metabolic*: obesity (lack of exercise with excessive calorie consumption is by far the commonest cause of weight gain in the world), pregnancy (the next commonest cause of progressive weight gain)
- *Endocrine*: cyclical weight changes relating to the menstrual cycle, menopause and premature ovarian failure (low oestrogen states), Cushing's syndrome (chronic exposure to corticosteroids), polycystic ovarian syndrome (PCOS), hypothyroidism, Cushing's disease (a pituitary adenoma produces excessive adrenocorticotrophic hormone, which overstimulates the adrenal glands, which then produce excessive endogenous corticosteroids)
- *Causes of gross oedema*: heart failure, liver failure, renal failure, fluid overload
- *Psychiatric conditions*: atypical depression, binge eating disorder
- *Very rare causes of secondary obesity*: Prader–Willi syndrome (deletion of a portion of the long arm of chromosome 15), Lawrence–Moon–Biedl syndrome

History

History of presenting complaint
- Onset
  - Acute (heart failure, liver failure)
  - Subacute (hypothyroidism, PCOS, Cushing's disease, glucocorticoid excess, related to medications)

Medical Student Survival Skills: History Taking and Communication Skills, First Edition.
Philip Jevon and Steve Odogwu.
© 2020 John Wiley & Sons Ltd. Published 2020 by John Wiley & Sons Ltd.
Companion website: www.wiley.com/go/jevon/medicalstudent

- – Chronic (calorie excess, atypical depression, Prader–Willi syndrome)
- – Late (menopause)
- Time course
  - – Steadily progressive (pregnancy)
  - – Fluctuating (menstrual, binge eating disorder)
- Associated symptoms
  - – Otherwise well (calorie excess, pregnancy, menopause)
  - – Cold intolerance, diffuse hair loss, menorrhagia, poor concentration, fatigue, constipation (hypothyroidism)
  - – Central obesity, abdominal striae, poor wound healing, easy bruising, buffalo hump, proximal muscle weakness, fatigue (Cushing's disease)
  - – Hirsuitism, irregular periods, acne, greasy hair (PCOS)
  - – Low self-esteem, low mood, lack of energy, lack of enjoyment, avoidance of social eating situations, consumption of large amounts of food followed by self-punishing behaviours (depression, binge eating disorder)
  - – Breathlessness, orthopnoea, paroxysmal nocturnal dyspnoea, chest pain, poor exercise tolerance, lower limb swelling (heart failure)
  - – Jaundice, abdominal swelling, unsteadiness, tremor, itching (liver failure)
  - – Malaise, fatigue, itching, abdominal aching (renal failure)

Past medical history
- Ask about complications of obesity:
  - – Diabetes
  - – Heart disease
  - – Cerebrovascular disease
  - – Joint disease
  - – Fatty liver and cirrhosis
  - – Varicose veins
  - – Hernias
  - – Sleep apnoea and pulmonary hypertension
- Ask about conditions that may point to the cause of obesity:
  - – Chronic dermatoses, rheumatoid arthritis, chronic obstructive pulmonary disease, inflammatory bowel disease, severe asthma (steroid use)
  - – Depression, psychoses (antidepressant and antipsychotic use)
  - – Angina, myocardial infarction, high blood pressure, high cholesterol (heart failure, use of beta-blockers)

Medications and allergies
- Corticosteroids (prednisolone)
- Antidepressants (selective serotonin reuptake inhibitors, e.g. fluoxetine, and paroxetine; tricyclics, e.g. amitriptyline)
- Anticonvulsants (valproate)
- Antipsychotics (olanzapine, chlorpromazine)
- Beta-blockers (propranolol, atenolol)
- Progesterone-based contraceptives (depot injection, 'mini-pill')
- Insulin (can cause weight gain, but more likely to cause local lipodystrophy [fibrosis of fat tissue])

Family history
- Environmental influences (diet, exercise, hobbies)
- Parental obesity

Social history
- Food and exercise diary
- Stopping smoking (loss of nicotine stimulation slows metabolic rate and affects eating behaviour)
- Excessive alcohol consumption

OSCE Key Learning Points

✔ Obesity is almost always the result of environmental and behavioural influences. However, it is important to consider the medical causes, as these may be readily treatable; in particular hypothyroidism and other endocrine disorders

 Common misinterpretations and pitfalls

Although it is a clinically important observation, avoid stating that a patient is 'obese' or has a 'large body habitus/BMI' at the bedside. This can be reserved for the post-OSCE viva.

73 Weight loss

Definition: Unintentional loss of body mass over weeks or months.

Differentials

- *Reduced intake*: psychiatric illness, alcoholism, malignancy, neurological diseases, personal neglect
- *Increased metabolism*: stress, increased activity, malignancy, diabetes, thyrotoxicosis, Addison's disease, infections especially tuberculosis (TB) or human immunodeficiency virus (HIV)
- *Absorption problems*: inflammatory bowel disease, malabsorption syndromes, coeliac disease, high output stoma
- *Iatrogenic*: diuretic use

History

 NB Infection control measures if you suspect infective causes.

History of presenting complaint
- Onset and duration of weight loss
- Amount of weight loss/clothes size change
- Associated symptoms
  - Nausea and vomiting
  - Recent change in diet or appetite
  - History of dysphagia
  - Regurgitation or heartburn

Medical Student Survival Skills: History Taking and Communication Skills, First Edition.
Philip Jevon and Steve Odogwu.
© 2020 John Wiley & Sons Ltd. Published 2020 by John Wiley & Sons Ltd.
Companion website: www.wiley.com/go/jevon/medicalstudent

- – Change in bowel habit especially diarrhoea, stool changes, mucus, blood (see Chapter 15)
- – Palpitations, heat intolerance, tremor, increased bowel frequency, noticed neck lump, anxiety
- – Dizziness (particularly postural), lethargy, skin pigmentation
- – Cough, fever, night sweats, recent travel
- – Polydipsia/polyuria
- – Red flags for malignancy
- History of confusion/dementia
- Fluid balance (intake/output)
- Personal perspective of body image or change in mood, concentration, and sleep

Past medical and surgical history
- History of any chronic diseases and symptoms of progression (e.g. in chronic obstructive pulmonary disease)
- History of malignancy
- History of dementia
- History of any abdominal surgery, particularly upper gastrointestinal
- Any other medical/surgical problems

Medications and allergies
- Use of over the counter diet medications
- Current medications especially digoxin, metformin and levodopa, diuretics
- Compliance with medications
- Allergy history

Family history
- History of malignancy, thyroid problems, diabetes, inflammatory bowel diseases
- Any medical conditions running in the family

Social history
- Who patient lives with
- Exercise habits, current mobility and ability to do activities of daily living
- Current housing situation – bungalow/stairs
- Occupation history
- Smoking and passive smoking history

- Recent travel
- Alcohol history and IV drug use
- Sexual health
- Do they need assistance in eating and, if so, is it available to them

OSCE Key Learning Points

✔ Weight loss is a red flag for malignancy and TB/HIV

 NB Do not forget about social reasons for weight loss; dementia can also cause people to lose weight.

 Common misinterpretations and pitfalls

- Anyone can get TB or HIV – do not make clinical decisions on stereotypes
- Weight loss can be a symptom of all chronic diseases – poor management of these diseases may cause weight loss

74 Wheeze

Definition: An abnormal respiratory sound heard as a result of narrowing of the lower airways.

A wheeze is usually heard in expiration, although it can occur in inspiration. It can be monophonic – signalling narrowing of a single airway. A polyphonic wheeze may indicate narrowing of multiple airways of different calibres.

Differentials

- *Common*: exacerbation of chronic obstructive pulmonary disease (COPD)/asthma, infective (pneumonia/bronchitis), acute left ventricular failure
- *Rare*: anaphylaxis, tumour, foreign body

History

 NB If there is an immediate airway threat, call for help.

History of presenting complaint
- Onset, duration, frequency
- Exacerbating/relieving factors – including diurnal variation
- Cough – productive, white/green/pink/bloody, frothy, nocturnal
- Shortness of breath (see Chapter 62)
- Fever, confusion
- Chest pain, palpitations, syncope, orthopnoea, paroxysmal nocturnal dyspnoea, leg swelling
- Eating unusual foods in past few hours, exposure to animals/chemicals

Medical Student Survival Skills: History Taking and Communication Skills, First Edition.
Philip Jevon and Steve Odogwu.
© 2020 John Wiley & Sons Ltd. Published 2020 by John Wiley & Sons Ltd.
Companion website: www.wiley.com/go/jevon/medicalstudent

- Facial swelling, itching, rash
- Weight loss, loss of appetite
- Exercise tolerance – normal and current

Past medical and surgical history
- History of asthma – if present consider if normal PEFR (peak expiratory flow rate), intensive care admissions
- History of COPD
- History of heart problems, e.g. ischaemic heart disease, valvular disease, congestive cardiac failure
- History of any other medical conditions or surgical procedures

Medications and allergies
- Current medications
- Compliance with medications
- Allergy history

Family history
- Asthma, heart disease
- Any medical conditions running in the family

Social history
- Who patient lives with – including pets
- Current mobility and ability to do activities of daily living
- Current housing situation – bungalow/stairs, damp/mould
- Occupation history – in particular miners, asbestos exposure, factory workers
- Smoking and passive smoking history
- Recent travel – air conditioning units (*Legionella*)
- Alcohol history

OSCE Key Learning Points

✔ Do not forget about cardiac causes of a wheeze

 NB A monophonic wheeze, history of weight loss, and smoking history should make you think about cancer.

Common misinterpretations and pitfalls

- Confusing a wheeze with stridor (stridor is an upper airway respiratory sound, usually inspiratory); stridor may indicate impending airway obstruction
- A wheeze can be serious, especially in asthmatics; do not be reassured if a wheeze suddenly stops in these patients

Part 2

Communication Skills

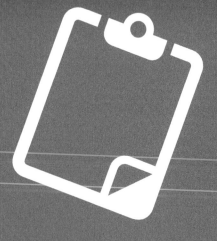

75 Alcohol advice

Alcohol can cause widespread harm to a person's health. In 2016, 81% of the UK population drank alcohol. In the same year, 31% of men and 16% of women reported that they drank above the recommended limits. Alcohol can not only affect people's health, but also their relationships and economic situation.

Definitions

- Increasing risk
  - Adults who regularly drink more than 14 units of alcohol a week
- High risk
  - Men who regularly drink ≥ 8 units a day
  - Women who regularly drink ≥ 6 units a day
- Alcohol dependence (ICD-10)
  - Strong desire to drink alcohol
  - Difficulty controlling use
  - Persistence in drinking alcohol despite the harm
  - Alcohol takes a higher priority in the person's life above other activities
  - Increased tolerance
  - Sometimes physical withdrawal
  - First thought on waking up is 'where is my next drink (alcohol)?'
- Recommended limits (2013)
  - Men should not regularly drink ≥ 3 units a day
  - Women should not regularly drink ≥ 2 units a day
  - Regularly = drinking these amounts every day/most days
- Units
  - 25 ml of spirits = 1 unit
  - Alcopop or can/bottle of regular lager = 1.5 units
  - Pint of regular beer/lager/cider = 2.5 units

Medical Student Survival Skills: History Taking and Communication Skills, First Edition.
Philip Jevon and Steve Odogwu.
© 2020 John Wiley & Sons Ltd. Published 2020 by John Wiley & Sons Ltd.
Companion website: www.wiley.com/go/jevon/medicalstudent

- 175 ml glass of wine = 2 units
- Bottle of wine = 9 units

 NB Ensure you are in a quiet room, and sit down with the patient if possible.

Alcohol History

- Do you drink alcohol?
  - How much alcohol do you drink a day/week/month?
- CAGE questionnaire (≥ 2 'yes' answers could indicate alcohol dependence):
  - Do you think you need to **C**ut down on your alcohol intake?
  - Does it **A**nnoy you when people criticise your drinking?
  - Do you feel **G**uilty about your drinking?
  - Do you need an (**E**ye opener) **E**arly morning drink to steady your nerves/rid a hangover?
- When do you drink alcohol?
- Are there any situations in which you feel you need to drink alcohol?
- Can you think of a reason why you drink alcohol?
- The FAST question 'How often do you drink eight or more drinks on one occasion?' detects 70% of hazardous drinkers if the answer is weekly or more often

Benefits of Cutting Down/Stopping

- Explain they are drinking above the recommended limits
- Explain the health benefits of cutting down/stopping drinking; alcohol can increase the risk of:
  - Dyspepsia, gastric bleeding
  - Liver disease
  - Pancreatitis (incidence higher in Asian men)
  - Alcohol does not improve sleep
  - Alcohol exacerbates depression which reduces or stops 4–6 weeks after stopping alcohol
  - Raised blood pressure
  - Irregular heartbeats
  - Coronary heart disease
  - Stroke

- Cancer of the mouth, oesophagus, and larynx
- Breast cancer in women
- Decreased fertility
- Anxiety, cognitive impairment, and occasional psychotic reactions may occur with excess alcohol use
- Explain the cost-benefits of cutting down/stopping drinking
  - Ask the patient how much they spend on alcohol, and calculate the amount that adds up to in a year
- Discuss the effects on family and friends of increased alcohol intake
- Discuss the effects on work of increased alcohol intake

How to Cut Down/Stop

This should be a discussion.
- Ask the patient if they feel they could cut down/stop drinking alcohol
  - Discuss with them various things they feel could help
- Emphasise that it is their responsibility to cut down/stop
- Offer them support
  - Repeat appointment
  - If appropriate, information on:
    - Addaction (www.addaction.org.uk), Alcoholics Anonymous (http://www.alcoholics-anonymous.org.uk), Drinkaware (www.drinkaware.co.uk)
    - Advice lines (e.g. Drink Line 0800 917 8282)
- Discuss goals/aims – daily/weekly targets
- Offer written information leaflets
- If a person is dependent, suddenly stopping all alcohol can lead to seizures. It is counterintuitive, but recommend that they reduce their intake and do not stop suddenly

Advice for Family Members/Friends

- Family members may attend worrying about a relative's drinking
- Advise them to:
  - Talk to the person they are worried about (when the person is sober and they are calm)
  - Listen to the person they are worried about – avoid arguments
  - Explain what problems the drinking is causing
  - Be consistent

- Be clear about what they want to the person that they are worried about
- Seek support from family/friends/websites/advice lines
- Be realistic and encourage the person they are worried about to be realistic
- Do not aid the person's addiction
- Remind them that it is dangerous to suddenly stop all alcohol if the person is dependent
- Explain the person they are worried about will only stop drinking if they want to. If the person is dependent on alcohol it can be very difficult for them to stop drinking and they may need professional support
- A dependent drinker's behaviour is completely ruled by the need for more alcohol
- Try to find something the person can like about themselves or be proud of, e.g. admitting they have a problem in the first place
- Detoxing from alcohol with the aid of medication can be dangerous and should be done after careful assessment by a healthcare professional skilled in this area and the person should be admitted to a unit or have the support of family members

OSCE Key Learning Points

✔ Giving alcohol advice can be challenging
✔ Learn the recommended limits of alcohol
✔ Not all the points need to be covered in one session, be guided by the patient about what is important to them

 NB There are many different tools to assess a patient's drinking: the CAGE questionnaire, the short three question audit (Audit-C), and the full 10 question audit (Audit-10) are the common ones.

Common misinterpretations and pitfalls

Do not be judgemental. Anyone can have alcohol dependence, no matter their background. It is important to discuss alcohol with all patients. It has been shown that identification and brief advice can be effective. If the patient drinks heavily then advise them *not* to stop drinking suddenly.

76 The angry patient

Dealing with angry patients or relatives is a difficult task for everyone. Effective communication skills can often defuse the situation and lead to effective dialogue with the patient or relative. Patients and/or relatives can become angry for a variety of reasons.

Causes

- Long wait to see a healthcare professional
- Bad news
- Expectations were not met
- They feel as though they have lost control
- Personality disorders/substance abuse/anxiety/alcohol/drugs
- An error has been made or has been perceived to be made
- They feel as though they have no other options
- A delay or perceived delay in treatment/diagnosis

Warning Signs

- Raised voice
- Abusive language
- Threatening language
- Red faced
- Loss of eye contact
- Clenched jaw
- Tense posture
- Clenched fists
- Fidgeting
- Invading personal space

Medical Student Survival Skills: History Taking and Communication Skills, First Edition.
Philip Jevon and Steve Odogwu.
© 2020 John Wiley & Sons Ltd. Published 2020 by John Wiley & Sons Ltd.
Companion website: www.wiley.com/go/jevon/medicalstudent

Dos

- Be prepared
- Think about the location of the consultation – such as exit routes/alarms
- Remain calm
- Talk in a soft, calm voice
- Keep a safe distance
- Express concern as to the cause of their anger – empathise
- Acknowledge why they are angry
- Encourage the patient to explain why they are angry
- Discuss what action they would like to be taken
- If appropriate, offer to take action
- Bring the consultation back to the reason you are there
- If the situation has escalated too far – your safety is paramount – *get out*

Don'ts

- Raise your voice
- Blame others
- Be confrontational
- Ignore the patient
- Invade their space
- Fuel the patient's anger

OSCE Key Learning Points

✔ Remaining calm is paramount, showing your own anger is not helpful.

 NB If the situation has escalated too far – your safety is paramount – *get out*

Common misinterpretations and pitfalls

Patients often become angry as a response to another emotion such as frustration/sadness/shock. It is important to address these emotions.

77 Breaking bad news or results

Before the Investigation

The patient should be counselled about the possible results of any tests, and about the course of action after the investigation results are available. For example, the need for potential invasive investigations after cancer screening, and the implications of possible negative or positive results.

Preparing to Give the Result

Do research
- Know what the results mean and be able to explain them in layman's terms
- Understand the next steps in investigations/treatment – including palliation
  - E.g. too advanced to cure but can treat the symptoms
- Be aware of the socioeconomic implications of diagnosis/management and be able to give correct advice
  - E.g. driving, time off work, childcare, implications if they are a carer for someone else (e.g. having to keep a minimum distance after radioactive treatment)
  - Specialist nurses are often able to give practical advice and signpost appropriate services
- Be aware of the implications of diagnosis on other family members and contacts
  - E.g. if they need to be investigated for infectious diseases/genetic conditions

Give them enough time
- Book a long appointment slot
- Turn off bleep/mobile phone or hand to a colleague

Medical Student Survival Skills: History Taking and Communication Skills, First Edition.
Philip Jevon and Steve Odogwu.
© 2020 John Wiley & Sons Ltd. Published 2020 by John Wiley & Sons Ltd.
Companion website: www.wiley.com/go/jevon/medicalstudent

Find an appropriate room
- The room should be quiet
- There should be enough space to sit down
- Make it clear to other staff that the room is not to be disturbed

Delivering the Results

- If results are abnormal or the news is bad, give warning shots, for example:
  - 'Have you got anyone that you'd like to bring in?'
  - 'I'm afraid that these are not the results that we were hoping for'.
- If the results are normal – explain that they may need further investigations or screening later in life; a negative result now does not mean that they will not contract the disease in the future
- Give at least a minute's silence
- Ask open questions
- Respond to emotional reactions, for example:
  - 'I can see that you are upset; what is worrying you the most?'
- Give written information – they are unlikely to retain much information
- Arrange appropriate follow-up
  - Soon
  - Be aware that much information will need to be repeated
  - Encourage them to write down questions to bring in next time
  - Provide a telephone number/method of contacting services if necessary before the next appointment

78 The deaf patient

One in seven people in the UK have some form of hearing loss. Hearing loss can range from complete loss of hearing to a mild hearing impairment. The patient may have been born deaf, or developed hearing loss in later life. Patients who use sign language usually have profound deafness. Sign language has its own punctuation and grammar. This should be considered when using written language.

Definitions

- *Mild deafness* (loss in range 25–39 dB):difficult to follow speech in noisy situations
- *Moderate deafness* (loss in range 40–69 dB): may need hearing aids
- *Severe deafness* (loss in range 70–94 dB): may need hearing aids, may use lip reading, sign language may be preferred language
- *Profound deafness* (loss in range ≥95 dB): sign language is likely to be preferred language
- The use of the word 'Deaf' with a capital D suggests the patient considers themselves a part of the Deaf community and uses sign language

 NB Think about the environment; arrange the room in an appropriate manner and minimise background noise.

Communication

- If possible, ask the patient their preferred communication style
- Face the patient
- Ensure the patient is looking at you
- Speak clearly

Medical Student Survival Skills: History Taking and Communication Skills, First Edition.
Philip Jevon and Steve Odogwu.
© 2020 John Wiley & Sons Ltd. Published 2020 by John Wiley & Sons Ltd.
Companion website: www.wiley.com/go/jevon/medicalstudent

- Do not shout
- Do not over exaggerate lip movements – it makes it difficult to lip read
- Ensure good lighting
- Do not cover your mouth
- Signpost the consultation:
  - 'Now we will talk about …' 'Now I will examine you …'
- If you are not understood, try re-phrasing the question
- Ask open ended questions
- Ask the patient to summarise what you have told them in order to gauge if you have been understood
- If examining the patient, explain clearly what you are going to do

The Patient Who Can Use British Sign Language

- Patients will often bring a family member/friend who can use sign language. However, it is always better to have a proper interpreter as they are trained and the patient/friend/relative can be saved from embarrassment when talking about sensitive topics. Use of an official interpreter also avoids bias in the interpretation
- Use a fully accredited interpreter
- If using an interpreter, ensure that the patient can see both you and the interpreter
- Face the patient
- Talk to the patient

OSCE Key Learning Points

✔ It is your responsibility to ensure effective communication. Without this a patient may feel anxious, take medication incorrectly, or be unable to give an informed consent to treatment. It may also lead to an incorrect diagnosis

 NB For patients who use sign language – written communication may be useful for a brief interaction, but is not useful for a full consultation.

Common misinterpretations and pitfalls

- Do not assume the patient understands simply because they nod or say yes
- Do not assume that because a patient cannot hear you they are not competent. You should make every effort to ensure effective communication

79 Diabetes counselling

Management

Non-medical
- Life style changes – to reduce deterioration of diabetes and reduce the risk of cardiovascular disease:
  - Low sugar diet
  - Stop smoking
  - Healthy weight
  - Reduce alcohol consumption – risk of hypoglycaemia
- Education course – about condition and specific dietetic courses
- Importance of foot care
- Regular sight tests
- Annual diabetes review by GP or hospital

Medical
- Type 1 diabetics – insulin
- Type 2 diabetics – oral medication with progression onto subcutaneous medication and insulin if poorly controlled
- Monitoring and good control of hypertension and renal function
- Up to date with immunisations (including annual influenza jab)

Target Ranges

- Capillary blood glucose (CBG)
  - Pre-meal: 4–7 mmol l^{-1}
  - Post-meal: < 10 mmol l^{-1}
- HbA1c: < 48 mmol l^{-1} (6.5%) – higher target if patient is at risk of hypoglycaemia

Medical Student Survival Skills: History Taking and Communication Skills, First Edition.
Philip Jevon and Steve Odogwu.
© 2020 John Wiley & Sons Ltd. Published 2020 by John Wiley & Sons Ltd.
Companion website: www.wiley.com/go/jevon/medicalstudent

- Triglyceride: $< 4.5 \, mmol \, l^{-1}$
- Blood pressure: $< 140/80 \, mmgHg$ (or $< 130/80 \, mmHg$ if there is end-organ damage)

Complications

Short-term hyperglycaemia

- CBG $> 15 \, mmol \, l^{-1}$
- Diabetic ketoacidosis (DKA)
- Hyperosmolar hyperglycaemic state (HHS)

Triggers
- Missed/reduced dose of medication/insulin
- Consumption of sugary/high carbohydrate food (e.g. overtreatment of hypoglycaemia)
- Illness/infection

Symptoms
- Thirst
- Blurred vision
- Abdominal pain, nausea, and vomiting
- Collapse

Treatment
- Follow sick day rules (Box 79.1)
- DKA and HHS are potentially life-threatening
- Seek medical attention if:
  - Ketones in urine (type 1 diabetics only)
  - Unable to eat/drink and CBGs remain high

Box 79.1 Sick day rules (may vary between NHS Trusts)

- Continue with insulin, even if not eating or if vomiting – seek medical help if unable to eat/drink and CBGs are high
- Check CBG regularly and increase insulin if necessary – including at night
- Check for urinary or capillary ketones – seek medical help if present
- Drink lots of sugar-free drinks
- Continue to eat as much as possible; carbohydrates especially

Long-term hyperglycaemia

- *Macrovascular* – increased risk of stroke, myocardial infarction, and peripheral vascular disease
- *Microvascular* – retinopathy, neuropathy, nephropathy

Hypoglycaemia

- CBG $< 4\,mmol\,l^{-1}$

Triggers (sometimes unclear)
- Missed meal
- Too much insulin/certain medication
- Unexpected exertion
- Consumption of large quantity of alcohol or drinking alcohol without food

Symptoms (variable between patients)
- Sweating
- Shaking
- Hunger
- Irritability/change in mood, lack of concentration
- Blurred vision

Treatment
- Check CBG if able to/not too unwell
- Ingest short-acting and long-acting carbohydrates
- Recheck CBG after 5–10 minutes
- If patient unable to swallow, urgent treatment may be required with parenteral options (e.g. IM glucagon, or IV glucose)

Driving

The Law
- Group 1 drivers (cars and motorbikes) must notify the DVLA (Driver and Vehicle Licensing Agency) if they are:
  - On insulin
  - On non-insulin medication and have experienced severe hypoglycaemia (i.e. dependent on others for treatment, two episodes in past year), or have experienced hypoglycaemia whilst driving, or have developed reduced awareness
- Group 2 drivers (bus or lorry):
  - Must notify the DVLA if they are on any medication for diabetes
  - Will require annual medical assessment

Advice
- Check CBG within 2 hours before a car journey
- Stop for regular breaks to check CBG and eat (at least every 2 hours if on insulin)
- Keep short-acting and long-acting carbohydrate snacks in the car at all times
- If you develop symptoms of hypoglycaemia or feel unwell:
  - Pull over
  - Remove keys
  - Move to passenger seat
  - Check CBG – if low have fast- and long-acting carbohydrate snacks and do not start driving until the CBG is normal for at least 45 minutes

80 Explaining a clinical procedure

Background

Patients have a right to make informed, autonomous (where possible) decisions about their treatment and to be informed of the risks, benefits, and alternatives to their planned treatment. In order to treat patients, we must obtain their *consent*.

Consent

The process by which a patient makes an informed decision as to whether investigations and/or treatment will take place. Consent for a procedure should only be obtained by an individual competent in performing the intended procedure.

Discussing a Procedure

- Name of the proposed procedure
  - Explain as simply as possible, e.g. instead of 'laprascopic cholecystectomy' say 'removal of the gall bladder via keyhole surgery'
- The name of the person(s) responsible for the procedure
- An explanation of what the procedure will involve
- An explanation of the intended benefits
- An explanation of the serious or frequently occurring risks
  - Examples of common risks include pain, bleeding, infection, scar formation, wound breakdown, need for further surgery/procedure
  - Any risk that carries severe or life-altering consequences for the patient (e.g. stoma formation during bowel surgery, loss of motor function/sensation during ENT surgery close to the facial nerve) *regardless* of frequency
- A discussion about any additional procedures that may become necessary during the intended treatment e.g. blood transfusion, conversion of laprascopic procedure to laparotomy

Medical Student Survival Skills: History Taking and Communication Skills, First Edition.
Philip Jevon and Steve Odogwu.
© 2020 John Wiley & Sons Ltd. Published 2020 by John Wiley & Sons Ltd.
Companion website: www.wiley.com/go/jevon/medicalstudent

- There is no formal law dictating what a common or serious risk is. Information should be communicated in accordance to best practice (the Bolam test). A useful rule of thumb is to consider risks that occur in *1% of cases or greater to be frequently occurring.*
- Patients should be given time to ask questions and to consider information before deciding whether or not to give their consent to treatment.
- When discussing an intervention, it is important to address a patient's need, wishes, and priorities. Information should be conveyed according to their level of knowledge and understanding of the condition. *No assumptions* should be made regarding what a patient may want or need. Patients should be given information to a reasonable standard, but any information they directly request should be provided.

OSCE Key Learning Points

✔ Use as simple language as possible
✔ Be very clear about what the procedure involves, who will be doing it, and who is responsible
✔ Be blunt when discussing risks – it is essential the patient knows about them!
✔ Ensure the patient has time to weigh up the information and has enough time to ask you any questions

81 Insulin counselling

Insulin is made naturally in the body to push glucose from the blood into body cells to use for energy. There are three main groups of insulin:
- Animal
- Human – not from a human, but a synthetic molecule like human insulin
- Analogue – a molecule similar to insulin

Types of Insulin

There are six main types of insulin, which work in different ways (Table 81.1).

Timing

There are different injecting regimes, including:
- Once daily
- Twice daily
- Basal bolus
- Continuous infusion/insulin pump

Insulin regimes are chosen and tailored to the patient by the patient and their healthcare team.

Storage of Insulin

- Insulin needs to be kept below $25\,°C$; between 2 and $6\,°C$ is ideal (e.g. in a fridge)
- Insulin should be disposed of if it has been out of the fridge for more than 28 days

Medical Student Survival Skills: History Taking and Communication Skills, First Edition.
Philip Jevon and Steve Odogwu.
© 2020 John Wiley & Sons Ltd. Published 2020 by John Wiley & Sons Ltd.
Companion website: www.wiley.com/go/jevon/medicalstudent

Table 81.1 Types of insulin

Type of insulin	Peak of action	Duration of action
Rapid-acting analogue	0–30 minutes	2–5 hours
Long-acting analogue	No peak	24 hours
Short-acting insulin	2–6 hours	8 hours
Medium- and long-acting insulin	4–12 hours	30 hours
Mixed insulin Medium- and short-acting insulin	–	–
Mixed analogue Medium-acting insulin and rapid-acting analogue	–	–

Administration

- The insulin is injected into a fatty area where it gets absorbed into the body
  - The most common sites are the thighs, stomach, and buttocks
  - Sometimes other sites are recommended
- The needle is very small and, although it may be slightly painful initially, injecting should become easier
- It is important to change where you inject in a particular site to avoid getting lumps under the skin (called lipohypertrophy)

Discarding Needles

- Needles need to be disposed of correctly to prevent injury to the patient and others
- Disposal equipment (e.g. sharps bins) are provided on prescription and each local area will provide guidance on methods of disposal

Special Circumstances

- A patient should only withhold their normal insulin if their capillary blood glucose (CBG) is low
- Insulin should be continued, and increased if necessary, when ill, even if not eating or vomiting as illness can cause hyperglycaemia

82 Life style advice post myocardial infarction

Before counselling

- Introduce yourself and gain consent
- Explain the importance of secondary prevention following myocardial infarction (MI) in reducing the risk of subsequent MI

Counselling session

Improving diet
- Discuss current diet
- Advise a Mediterranean-style diet
- Two to four portions of oily fish per week (omega-3)
- Reduce simple carbohydrates intake
- Increase complex carbohydrates intake
- Encourage the patient to maintain a healthy weight

Alcohol intake
- Determine current intake
- Avoid binge drinking
- Safe limits:
  - Adults should consume no more than 14 units per week

Exercise
- Determine current level of exercise
- 20–30 minutes of exercise a day

Medical Student Survival Skills: History Taking and Communication Skills, First Edition.
Philip Jevon and Steve Odogwu.
© 2020 John Wiley & Sons Ltd. Published 2020 by John Wiley & Sons Ltd.
Companion website: www.wiley.com/go/jevon/medicalstudent

- Increase intensity and capacity gradually
- If prescribed glyceryl trinitrate (GTN) take it prior to exercise

Smoking cessation
- Encourage smokers to stop
- Offer those willing to stop support, leaflets, and referral

Going back to work
- Most people return to work 4–6 weeks after an MI
- If in a heavy manual job – return to work may take longer

Sexual activity
- Reassure that it is safe to resume sexual activity
- Sexual activity can be resumed when the patient has recovered and is comfortable (approximately 4 weeks)

Medications
- Encourage patients to comply with medications
- Ensure there are no interactions between medications, e.g. advise patient not to take PDE-5 inhibitors (sildenafil) if using GTN

Driving
- Stop driving for at least 1 month post MI
- Patient may need to inform the DVLA (Driver and Vehicle Licensing Agency) if they drive a large goods vehicle (LGV) or passenger carrying vehicle (PGV)

Flying
- Uncomplicated recovery – safe to fly after 2–3 weeks
- Seek advice from clinician about flying

Chest pain
- What to do if the patient gets chest pain, including resting, the use of GTN, and when to call 999 for the ambulance service

After counselling

- Allow opportunity for patient to ask questions
- Avoid using jargon
- Offer the patient an information leaflet

83 Cessation of smoking

Take a Short History

Smoking history
- What are they currently smoking – cigarettes or roll-ups
- How many are they smoking per day – has this increased or decreased
- How long have they been a smoker
- What reasons do they give or what appeals to them about quitting smoking
- Have they tried to stop smoking previously, which method did they use
- If it failed, after how long and what led to them restarting smoking
- Did they have any withdrawal symptoms

Social history
- Occupation
- Stressful job/home life
- Alcohol intake

Communication

Initially congratulate the patient on deciding to quit smoking. This may have been a very difficult decision for them to make.

- Establish what their ideas, concerns, and expectations are on quitting smoking
- Provide them with background information and the dangers of smoking

For example: Cigarettes contain nicotine. After smoking regularly for a period of time, the body gets used to nicotine supply and your body begins to depend on it. Tobacco smoke contains about 4000 chemicals, of which nicotine is just one. Other poisons taken in by smoking are tar, carbon monoxide (found also in car exhaust fumes), ammonia (used in floor cleaner), and arsenic (used in rat poison). At least 40 of the chemicals in tobacco smoke are proven to cause cancers of the lung, throat, mouth, bladder, and kidneys and the smoke also causes a number of other cancers.

Medical Student Survival Skills: History Taking and Communication Skills, First Edition.
Philip Jevon and Steve Odogwu.
© 2020 John Wiley & Sons Ltd. Published 2020 by John Wiley & Sons Ltd.
Companion website: www.wiley.com/go/jevon/medicalstudent

How to Quit Smoking

- Go cold turkey – make a date and stop completely
- Get rid of anything that reminds you of smoking, e.g. ashtrays
- Do not start when there are potentially stressful events coming up
- Get a friend or family member involved – support and motivation for both of you to stop
- Write down a list of reasons why you want to stop and get these out when you have strong cravings – you will need this to motivate you
- Think of some distraction techniques such as a new hobby – e.g. jogging, cooking. Be aware of eating as a distraction method as this is why people find they start to gain weight and then restart smoking
- Think of ways for dealing with people or places where you used to enjoy smoking, e.g. at the pub
- Get support by seeing the GP, get involved in a smoke-free group, see the website for information and support (see later in this chapter)
- There will be some blips but be ready for these and start again

Methods of Quitting Smoking

- Champix tablets (varenicline)
- Zyban tablets (bupropion)
- Nicotine replacement therapy

Champix and Zyban

Champix and Zyban tablets are for patients aged over 18 years old and are available on prescription only. You start taking them around 2 weeks before you want to quit smoking. Zyban works to reduce the withdrawal cravings you get after quitting smoking. Champix works to reduce the withdrawal cravings and reduces the feelings/effect that having a cigarette does to the body, making it easier to quit smoking. For both medications the patient should complete a 12 week course in total. They are not suitable in pregnancy and some health conditions.

Nicotine Replacement Therapy

There are six methods of taking nicotine replacement therapy.

- *Nicotine gum* is available in strengths and to start off with is taken every hour. It gives a small burst of nicotine as it absorbed through the lining off the mouth. It is most suitable for people who smoke more than 20 a day or are strongly addicted to nicotine

- *Microtabs* are small tablets that dissolve quickly under the tongue, giving short burst of nicotine. You should take one to two of these small tablets every hour when you first quit and then reduce down when ready
- *Lozenges* –are put in the mouth and take 20–30 minutes to dissolve, giving a slow release of nicotine. Initially you suck the lozenge to get nicotine; afterwards you can out it inside the cheek to continue releasing nicotine until it completely dissolves. When you first quit you should have one lozenge every 1–2 hours
- *Nicotine patches* are patches on the skin and come in different strengths depending on how much you smoke. They can last 16 hours or 24 hours. The patches release nicotine through the skin and directly into the blood stream. They are good if you want to stop smoking discreetly and do not like the taste of nicotine gum and lozenges
- *Nicotine inhalers* – look like plastic cigarettes and work best for people who will miss the feeling of having a cigarette in their hand. They work to release nicotine as a vapour which then gets absorbed through the mouth and throat. Inhalers work very quickly so when you have strong cravings for a cigarette you can reach for the inhaler

 NB Lozenges, inhalers, and nasal sprays should be used for a total of 12 weeks before stopping. Some patients will stop treatment too soon and then have urges to start smoking again.

- *Nicotine nasal sprays* –are sprayed into the nose and give the fastest and most effective dose of nicotine through the lining of nose. Each dose gives you the same amount of nicotine found in one cigarette. You should aim to spray once in each nostril every half an hour. It can be used a maximum of five times in 1 hour. Due to its fast-acting method it closely mimics the action of a normal cigarette and is therefore good for heavy smokers and smokers who have failed with other methods.

Some patients will state that some of the methods did not work for them and this is important as they may have not been on the correct dose for the amount they were smoking a day. You can advise the same method at a different dose or alternative methods. Encourage the patient if the current method is not working to get in touch to have the dose adjusted or try another method and not to give up. Make them aware it is a long process and they will not be able to stop smoking completely in just 2 weeks.

Things Offered on the NHS Website

- Support materials, advice, and different methods for quitting smoking
- Addiction test: – seven short questions to identify how addicted you are to nicotine. It gives you results with advice on what smoking methods will suit you best
- Quit Kit: a kit posted to your home with short tips and advice and tools to help with cravings
- A way of calculating the money you will save when you quit smoking and the effects smoking has on your body
- An online advisor if you are struggling and need to talk to someone as well as other useful contact numbers and support on your mobile phone

OSCE Key Learning Points

✔ Always be positive when a patient has reached for help and support to give up an addiction
✔ Ask about their ideas, concerns, and expectation of stopping smoking
✔ Be aware of the key points and methods to help them quit smoking
✔ Discuss distraction techniques
✔ Summarise and reinforce the health and financial benefits of stopping smoking
✔ Offer written information and signpost to the GP and internet

84 Oral steroids counselling

Types of Medication

Oral steroid are either glucocorticoids or mineralocorticoids (Table 84.1).

Advice to Patients

Before taking steroids
- Advise patient to read the patient information leaflet
- Patients must advise any healthcare professional treating them that they are on oral steroids
- Patients should keep the 'blue steroid card' available at all times

How to take steroids
- Take dose as prescribed by the doctor
- To be taken first thing in the morning with or after food (unless gastro-resistant tablets) in order to mimic circadian rhythm
- Remember to take the medication at the same time each day

Immunosuppression
- Increased susceptibility to infections, serious infections may go unnoticed
- Unless already immune, patients are at risk of severe chicken pox and measles, and so should avoid close contact

Adrenal suppression
- If corticosteroid treatment is given for more than 3 weeks, it must not be stopped abruptly
  - Long-term steroids should be stopped gradually over a few weeks to allow endogenous steroid production to recommence

Medical Student Survival Skills: History Taking and Communication Skills, First Edition.
Philip Jevon and Steve Odogwu.
© 2020 John Wiley & Sons Ltd. Published 2020 by John Wiley & Sons Ltd.
Companion website: www.wiley.com/go/jevon/medicalstudent

Table 84.1 Different oral steroids

Glucocorticoid (immunological and metabolic effects)	Mineralocorticoid (sodium and water retention)
Prednisolone	Cortisone
Prednisone	Hydrocortisone
Betamethasone	Fludrocortisone
Dexamethasone	
Deflazacort	

- Adrenal suppression may continue for up to a year or more after stopping treatment
- Patients should mention their course of steroid treatment when receiving treatment for any illness or injury

Mood and behaviour changes
- High doses in particular can alter mood and behaviour in the early stages (affects about five in every 100)
  - Confusion, irritability, delusional thoughts and in extremes cases thinking about suicide or having manic thoughts
- Seek medical advice if worrying psychological effects occur

Other serious effects
- Musculoskeletal side effects – osteoporosis
- Gastrointestinal effects – gastric and duodenal ulcers, oral thrush
- Ophthalmic effects – glaucoma, cataracts, thinning of the sclera
- Growth restriction in children and adolescents
- Metabolic effects – raising blood sugars, redistribution of body fat

If a dose is forgotten
- Advise patient to take it as soon as they remember if it is the same day
- If it is the following day, to take it at the time they would *normally* take the medication
- Never have more than one dose in the same day

OSCE Key Learning Points

✔ Long-term steroids should be gradually stopped to allow endogenous steroid production to recommence and avoid an adrenal crisis

✔ Ensure the patient is provided with a 'blue steroid card' to present to all persons involved in their care

✔ Advise patients of the mental health effects associated with steroids, and to report any changes in mood to the prescriber immediately

 NB Remember that high dose inhaled steroids used long term have significant systemic side effects similar to oral steroids.

Index

Note: Page numbers in **bold** refer to tables.

Medical Student Survival Skills: History Taking and Communication Skills, First Edition.
Philip Jevon and Steve Odogwu.
© 2020 John Wiley & Sons Ltd. Published 2020 by John Wiley & Sons Ltd.
Companion website: www.wiley.com/go/jevon/medicalstudent